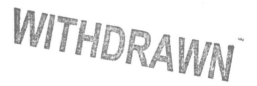

THE HIPPOCRATIC OATH AND
THE ETHICS OF MEDICINE

I SWEAR BY APOLLO THE PHYSICIAN AND BY ASCLEPIUS AND BY HEALTH [THE GOD HYGIEIA] AND PANACEA AND BY ALL THE GODS AS WELL AS GODDESSES, MAKING THEM JUDGES [WITNESSES], TO BRING THE FOLLOWING OATH AND WRITTEN COVENANT TO FULFILLMENT, IN ACCORDANCE WITH MY POWER AND MY JUDGMENT; TO REGARD HIM WHO HAS TAUGHT ME THIS TECHNÉ [ART AND SCIENCE] AS EQUAL TO MY PARENTS, AND TO SHARE, IN PARTNERSHIP, MY LIVELIHOOD WITH HIM AND TO GIVE HIM A SHARE WHEN HE IS IN NEED OF NECESSITIES, AND TO JUDGE THE OFFSPRING [COMING] FROM HIM EQUAL TO [MY] MALE SIBLINGS, AND TO TEACH THEM THIS TECHNÉ, SHOULD THEY DESIRE TO LEARN [IT], WITHOUT FEE AND WRITTEN COVENANT,AND TO GIVE A SHARE BOTH OF RULES AND OF LECTURES, AND OF ALL THE REST OF LEARNING, TO MY SONS AND TO THE [SONS] OF HIM WHO HAS TAUGHT ME AND TO THE PUPILS WHO HAVE BOTH MADE A WRITTEN CONTRACT AND SWORN BY A MEDICAL CONVENTION BUT BY NO OTHER.AND I WILL USE REGIMENS FOR THE BENEFIT OF THE ILL IN ACCORDANCE WITH MY ABILITY AND MY JUDGMENT, BUT FROM [WHAT IS] TO THEIR HARM OR INJUSTICE I WILL KEEP [THEM]. AND I WILL NOT GIVE A DRUG THAT IS DEADLY TO ANYONE IF ASKED [FOR IT], NOR WILL I SUGGEST THE WAY TO SUCH A COUNSEL. AND LIKEWISE I WILL NOT GIVE A WOMAN A DESTRUCTIVE PESSARY. AND IN A PURE AND HOLY WAY I WILL GUARD MY LIFE AND MY TECHNÉ. I WILL NOT CUT, AND CERTAINLY NOT THOSE SUFFERING FROM STONE, BUT I WILL CEDE [THIS] TO MEN [WHO ARE] PRACTITIONERS OF THIS ACTIVITY. INTO AS MANY HOUSES AS I MAY ENTER, I WILL GO FOR THE BENEFIT OF THE ILL, WHILE BEING FAR FROM ALL VOLUNTARY AND DESTRUCTIVE INJUSTICE, ESPECIALLY FROM SEXUAL ACTS BOTH UPON WOMEN'S BODIES AND UPON MEN'S, BOTH OF THE FREE AND OF THE SLAVES.AND ABOUT WHATEVER I MAY SEE OR HEAR IN TREATMENT, OR EVEN WITHOUT TREATMENT, IN THE LIFE OF HUMAN BEINGS — THINGS THAT SHOULD NOT EVER BE BLURTED OUT OUTSIDE —I WILL REMAIN SILENT, HOLDING SUCH THINGS TO BE UNUTTERABLE [SACRED, NOT TO BE DIVULGED].IF I RENDER THIS OATH FULFILLED, AND IF I DO NOT BLUR AND CONFOUND IT [MAKING IT TO NO EFFECT] MAY IT BE [GRANTED] TO ME TO ENJOY THE BENEFITS BOTH OF LIFE AND OF TECHN·, BEING HELD IN GOOD REPUTE AMONG ALL HUMAN BEINGS FOR TIME ETERNAL. IF, HOWEVER, I TRANSGRESS AND PERJURE MYSELF, THE OPPOSITE OF THESE.

THE HIPPOCRATIC OATH AND THE ETHICS OF MEDICINE

STEVEN H. MILES

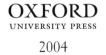

OXFORD
UNIVERSITY PRESS

2004

OXFORD
UNIVERSITY PRESS

Oxford   New York
Auckland   Bangkok   Buenos Aires   Cape Town   Chennai
Dar es Salaam   Delhi   Hong Kong   Istanbul   Karachi   Kolkata
Kuala Lumpur   Madrid   Melbourne   Mexico City   Mumbai
Nairobi   São Paulo   Shanghai   Taipei   Tokyo   Toronto

Copyright © 2004 by Oxford University Press, Inc.

Published by Oxford University Press, Inc.
198 Madison Avenue, New York, New York, 10016
http://www.oup-usa.org

Oxford is a registered trademark of Oxford University Press

Library of Congress Cataloging-in-Publication Data
Miles, Steven H.
The Hippocratic Oath and the ethics of medicine/
Steven H. Miles.
p. ; cm.
Includes bibliographical references and index
ISBN 0–19–516219–6
1. Hippocrates. Hippocratic oath.   2. Medical ethics.
3. Physicians — Professional ethics.
I. Title.
[DNLM: 1. Ethics, Medical.   2. Hippocratic Oath. W 50 M643t 2004]
R724.5.M54 2004
174'.22 — dc21   2003042954

2 4 6 8 9 7 5 3 1

Printed in the United States of America
on acid-free paper

PREFACE

This book was occasioned by a simple puzzle. While teaching a medical school seminar, I discovered that the students' translation of the Hippocratic Oath did not contain the word *injustice* while my translation used it twice. I set out to discover why this was so. This journey took me from many renditions of the *Oath*, to scholarship on it and other ancient Greek medical treatises, and to a widening exploration of Greek medicine and culture.

The *Oath* is the most admired work in Western European medical ethics. Like other icons, it is often venerated without question or understanding. In fairness, it is difficult to discern its meaning. It comes from an ancient culture that, though ancestral to ours, was very different. There are only a handful of substantial analyses of the *Oath* in the English language. Most are dated, technically written, and relatively inaccessible to the general reader.

This book examines the medical ethics of the *Oath*. It proceeds straightforwardly from beginning to end. Most commentators do not follow this seemingly obvious route. Many skim past words like "I swear by Apollo" that are laden with surprising meaning. Some focus on the modern concerns of euthanasia and abortion, thereby fashioning the *Oath's* passages on deadly drugs and destructive pessaries, which seem to have been merely illustrative examples of a principle, into its moral axis. Some rearrange passages according to thematic preferences. Such reconstructions obliterate the *Oath's* rhetorical and poetic structure.

The *Oath* was a composed discourse rather than an aggregation of promises bracketed by an opening invocation and a closing entreaty. Accordingly, I have divided this book into parts and chapters that follow its structure. The parts are sequences of passages that seem to form arguments in the larger composition. An introduction to each part discusses how and why the passages in that part seem to be linked to each other. Each ensuing chapter examines a specific passage from the *Oath*.

As a composition, the *Oath* implicitly posed, and explicitly answered, three questions. It answered the first question, Who are physicians? by tracing the lineage of healers back to Apollo, thereby pointing to myths that spoke to why and how humans heal and of the deference that physicians must give to the fact of human mortality. As the new medical apprentice swore to accept his physician-teacher as his father, he joined this lineage. It specified a physician's obligations to this family of teachers, colleagues, and medical descendents in a way that ensured the continuation of the professional lineage. It answered the second question, To what are physicians committed? with principles and rules that were organized into two stanzas: one addressed the ethic of physicians in society and the other addressed the physician in the clinical encounter. The third question, In what way are physicians accountable? was answered by defining the physician's commitment to the letter and the spirit of the *Oath* as evaluated by the larger human community. By saying that the human community ultimately judges physicians, the *Oath* invites our evaluation of its message.

Before we can consider the *Oath*'s meaning for our time, we must have some understanding of what it meant in its own time. This requires going to many kinds of sources. The foremost resources are the Greek medical writings of the fifth century BCE. Oddly enough, the ethics content of these documents has been offhandedly dismissed rather than examined. This is unfortunate because the context of the *Oath*'s words, "I will not give a deadly drug" can be clarified by looking at how Greek physicians cared for persons at the end of life and how they understood depression and suicide during severe illness. Works on ancient Greek anthropology, philosophy, and drama can also illuminate the mores and thinking of this time. With this deeper understanding, we can properly begin to satisfy our curiosity as to what the *Oath* might have to teach us.

We should not underestimate the difficulty of extrapolating ethics from such a different culture. The *Oath*'s core still rings true. Physicians are engaged in a moral enterprise secured by personal integrity and accountable to benefiting the ill and keeping them from injustice. However, the *Oath's* sense of medical ethics was shaped by its culture, including its acceptance of slavery and the subordinate status of women. The first chapter briefly describes the difficulty of using the *Oath* to speak to our time and offers several ways for understanding how the *Oath* has been invoked and applied to the medical ethics debates of today. Subsequent chapters close with true case vignettes (altered to guard confidentiality) to serve as illustrations for discussions of how much or how little can be done to bring the *Oath's* medical ethics forward. The Afterword offers some larger conclusions on what the *Oath* has of value for us.

This book focuses on the medical ethics of the *Oath*. It is not an encyclopedic exploration of ancient Greek medicine or of Greek medical ethics. The *Oath* does not discuss many issues in the medical ethics of its time. The status and rights of persons with mental illnesses or contagious diseases is not known. The role of public physicians deserves a fuller exploration. The Greek medical treatises on gynecology are only now being properly examined. Even so, the *Oath* can serve as an attractive and serviceable framework for a modern medical ethics curriculum rather than simply being relegated to ritualistic use. Appendix B shows how the *Oath* might be used to organize a medical ethics curriculum.

This book is for many kinds of readers. I hope that students in the health sciences will gain a better understanding of a text that they are likely to confront during their training. I hope clinicians will enjoy and benefit from this encounter with those who laid the foundation for Western medicine. I hope my colleagues in bioethics will acquire, as I have, an enhanced appreciation for Greek medical ethics. I hope general readers will enjoy this peek at an aspect of Greek culture. The main text is written to be accessible to all these audiences. A frontispiece map shows the places named throughout the book. A timeline in Appendix A lists major events, individuals, and the dates of ancient medical treatises. Appendix B is for those who teach medical ethics; it shows how the *Oath* can be used as a curricular outline. A bibliography is also provided with brief comments on the sources, a table of the confusing synonym titles for the Greek medical works, and a list of books that are repeatedly cited throughout this work. Endnotes contain citations and extended notes on topics of more specialized or speculative interest.

These readers might wonder what a physician–medical ethicist can bring to this topic. There are surprisingly few commentaries on the *Oath* as a whole. A rare exception is a twenty-page discussion by Leon Kass in his book, *Toward a More Natural Science* (1985). Before then, Ludwig Edelstein's 1943 article analyzed the *Oath* and proposed that Pythagorean philosophers wrote it, a view that current scholars now largely reject (see Chapter 3). Dr. Edelstein's work preceded the development of the modern field of bioethics, which Al Jonsen dates to about 1960. I have been privileged to teach and write in that field for twenty years. It has created new ways of articulating the moral dimensions of medical work. Such concepts can be used to reflect on the medical practice of ancient Greece. Studies of ancient Greek culture and its medical system have also greatly progressed since the work of Dr. Edelstein and even of Dr. Kass. For example, about twenty of the ancient Greek medical texts have been authoritatively translated into English during the last fifty years.

The *Oath* has not been examined in light of those medical treatises since Dr. Edelstein dismissed those works as merely containing bedside decorum. In fact, the ancient works described such matters as how the physicians of that time perceived and understood their patients, their attitudes toward death and abortions, how to talk with patients and secure their consent to treatment, fair marketplace competition for business, and many other issues. These matters are the substance of medical ethics today. Physicians from Galen to Kass have contributed to interpreting Greek medicine. As a practicing physician and medical ethicist, my primary work is to examine the *Oath* in light of the medical culture of its time while looking at the relationship between its view of medical ethics and possibly related issues for medicine in our time. The ancient manuscripts themselves are long gone. Very few scholars are qualified to assemble the variant texts that remain, reconcile their differences, and translate them into modern languages. I relied on those authoritative translations (see Bibliography). I read some of the French scholarship but am unable to read German scholars of ancient Greek medicine.

Many people shaped this work. I thank my colleagues at the Center for Bioethics at the University of Minnesota, especially Director Jeffrey Kahn, for encouraging and critiquing this work. Dr. Frank Cerra's administrative support for the Center for Bioethics has ensured a home for this scholarship. Many people offered helpful comments on various drafts, especially Howard Burchell, Al Jonsen, Nita Krevans, Mark Kuczewski, Kathryn Montgomery, Mischa Penn, Vivian Nutton, and my parents. The Soros Foundation's Project on Death in America provided substantial career development support. Remo Ostini,

Alicia Hall, William Vann, and the staff of the Owen H. Wangensteen Historical Library of Biology and Medicine helped me obtain many documents.
Catherine Zimba of For Goodness Graphics provided the map and timelines.
Morgan Grayce Willow provided editing assistance. Jeffrey House of Oxford
University Press is everything that an author could possibly ask of a publisher,
critic, and editor. Joline, Esmé, and Erica, my wife and daughters, are my strongest partners in everything I do.

Minneapolis, Minnesota   S.H.M.

CONTENTS

THE *OATH*[1]

I swear by Apollo the Physician and by Asclepius and by Health [the god Hygieia] and Panacea and by all the gods as well as goddesses, making them judges [witnesses], to bring the following oath and written covenant to fulfillment, in accordance with my power and my judgment;

to regard him who has taught me this techné[2] [art and science] as equal to my parents, and to share, in partnership, my livelihood with him and to give him a share when he is in need of necessities, and to judge the offspring [coming] from him equal to [my] male siblings, and to teach them this techné, should they desire to learn [it], without fee and written covenant,

and to give a share both of rules and of lectures, and of all the rest of learning, to my sons and to the [sons] of him who has taught me and to the pupils who have both made a written contract and sworn by a medical convention but by no other.

And I will use regimens for the benefit of the ill in accordance with my ability and my judgment, but from [what is] to their harm or injustice I will keep [them].

And I will not give a drug that is deadly to anyone if asked [for it], nor will I suggest the way to such a counsel.

And likewise I will not give a woman a destructive pessary.

And in a pure and holy way I will guard my life and my techné.

I will not cut, and certainly not those suffering from stone, but I will cede [this] to men [who are] practitioners of this activity.

Into as many houses as I may enter, I will go for the benefit of the ill, while being far from all voluntary and destructive injustice, especially from sexual acts both upon women's bodies and upon men's, both of the free and of the slaves.

And about whatever I may see or hear in treatment, or even without treatment, in the life of human beings—things that should not ever be blurted out outside—I will remain silent, holding such things to be unutterable [sacred, not to be divulged].

If I render this oath fulfilled, and if I do not blur and confound it [making it to no effect] may it be [granted] to me to enjoy the benefits both of life and of techné, being held in good repute among all human beings for time eternal. If, however, I transgress and perjure myself, the opposite of these.

NOTES

1. von Staden H. "In a pure and holy way": Personal and professional conduct in the Hippocratic Oath, J Hist Med Allied Sci 1996;51:406–8.

2 . *Techné* is defined in Chapter 8.

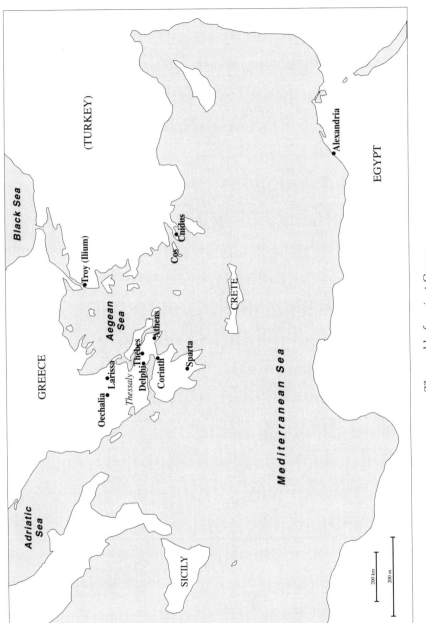

The world of ancient Greece.

THE HIPPOCRATIC OATH AND
THE ETHICS OF MEDICINE

1

GRAND ROUNDS

Rising faith in the promise of health-care technology and declining trust in the health-care system—such is the paradox of health care as the twenty-first century opens. Smallpox is extinct; polio is almost so. Lives are saved with seemingly miraculous transplants and chemotherapy. The ability to control high blood pressure is one of the many ways that modern health care prevents premature death or disability. Rehabilitation, prosthetics, and assistive devices enable persons with disabilities to live much better lives than they have in the past. In much of the world, infant mortality is falling and longevity is increasing.

Despite this cornucopia of treatments, mistrust haunts the public's and health professionals' view of the health-care system.[1] It is difficult for patients to trust physicians who are paid more by a health plan if they withhold costly tests or treatments.[2] It is difficult for the public to respect lavish medical centers that turn away children and adults without insurance. It is difficult to have confidence in researchers who are beholden to corporations that wish to advance their product and that design the studies, decide what data will be released, and even write up the results. It is difficult to admire a health-care system that reserves an undue portion of its best jobs for persons of privilege while the color of a patient's skin powerfully influences whether he or she will receive needed treatment for the pain of a broken bone or a diseased heart.

Patients and physicians alike want doctoring to be more than a job. I want my doctor to be as astute as Dr. Oliver Sacks and as altruistic as the medical missionary Albert Schweitzer. I want my doctor to be as all-around nice and accessible as television's Dr. Marcus Welby. I want a physician for whom medicine is more than a job, the kind of person who could swear an oath to uphold the highest possible professional aspirations.

Whatever happened to the Hippocratic Oath? After 2,400 years, its age is showing. It swears by Apollo and includes an ethic for treating slaves. It does not mention informed consent and disavows surgery. It did not anticipate managed care. Some say that its idea of one ethic for medicine is too idealistic. Others say we have fallen too far to aspire to its vision of good doctoring. Reading *Oath* might occasion a nostalgic reverie about the mythic nobility of medicine's ancient past or be a relaxing romp through history. Is it, however, relevant to medical ethics today?

One can deride *Oath* as "the ethical opiate of medicine." Often it is used as little more than a relic that is dusted off and recited at medical school ceremonies by students who have not seen it before and who will never see it again. Tiresome physicians wave it around like a censer in policy debates as they intone: "Trust us, we have the Hippocratic Oath and [insert the name of non-physician healers] do not." We have built up a tolerant disregard for the weight of its words.[3] Some say *Oath* articulates the moral essence of medicine, but often they stress particular passages, especially the ones on abortion and euthanasia, while skimming past others like the promise of free medical education for the sons of physicians. Such abuses notwithstanding, even if *Oath* is not *the* standard for good doctoring, it is *a* standard, and that makes it worth studying.

Aside from being a statement of medical ethics, *Oath* is a literary gem. At first glance, it reads like a simple Homeric oath: "I make a solemn promise. This is what I promise. Henceforth, judge me accordingly."[4] On closer inspection, its 400 words sweep from the mythic origin of medicine along a professional ancestry and point to the future human judgment on the profession. The *Oath* proposes principles and rules for medicine. These same words span the social order from gods to slaves.[5] In comparison with our endless rules for this and that, *Oath* seems elegantly complete. Was its time that much simpler, or was its author more stylish than our legalistic scriveners?

THE *OATH'S* MYSTERIOUS HISTORY

The Hippocratic Oath is an ancient Greek document that is simply entitled *Oath*. Its age is debated; 400 BCE is a reasonable estimate of when it was written.[6] That date is contemporaneous with the oldest of medical works written by generations of Greek physicians (see Appendix A). We do not know who composed it, and we do not know of any other document that appears to be by the same author. There is no evidence that Hippocrates wrote it, knew of it, or approved of it. There are no extant drafts or records of discussions of its terms. We do not know its stature in its own time or how widely or how long it was used. The *Oath* may be the only survivor of dozens of such oaths.

This lack of context for the *Oath* greatly complicates any effort to understand its meaning. The *Oath* is neither a sacred scripture nor a legal code. It appears to be designed for the swearing in of a person at the beginning of a medical apprenticeship. Essentially, the apprentice vows to repay his teachers and be a good physician in the manner described by the *Oath*. There are intense debates about the moral authority of the *Oath* in relation to the medical profession of its time. Scholars believe that few Greek physicians even knew of this oath, though the same is probably true of most of the ancient Greek medical texts. Most scholars do not believe that it represented the mainstream views of physicians in Greece of 400 BCE. Ludwig Edelstein asserts that ancient Greek physicians commonly performed euthanasia, abortion, and surgery and that the *Oath* reflected the views of a sect of philosophers rather than the medical ethics of the day (see Chapter 3). I believe that the *Oath* can be shown to be plausibly consonant with the medical practices and ethics of its time.

Part of the problem in understanding the relationship between the *Oath* and medical ethics is that the record of this relationship is nearly blank. The *Oath* was rarely mentioned during the first 1500 years of its existence. In the first century, Scribonius Largus referred to Hippocrates as the founder of the "calling [of medicine]" and to a single passage against abortion in a Hippocratic

Oath.[7] The oldest papyrus of the complete oath dates to 300 CE, about 700 years after it was written.[8] There are two citations of the *Oath* in the fourth century and two more from the fifth to eleventh centuries.[9] This paucity of references suggests that the *Oath* was neither widely used, nor influential, until the last 500 years or so. Medieval church scholars rediscovered it and began altering or interpreting it to conform to Christian doctrines in the Middle Ages.[10] From the eighteenth century onward, various versions of the *Oath* have been widely, though never universally, used in medical school graduation ceremonies in Europe and the United States.[11]

The *Oath* has been modified to serve a variety of purposes. Swearing by the Christian God rather than by Apollo was done at least a thousand years ago.[12] A very recent version for persons of all beliefs substitutes swearing by "whatever I hold sacred" for "I swear by Apollo." Parts were incorporated into a Hebrew medical oath in the fifth century CE.[13] During the last two hundred years, variants have been enlisted in support of charitable care and in opposition to abortion, euthanasia, physician-assisted suicide, torture, advertising of physicians' services, prescribing by psychologists,[14] and universal health care. New renditions are still being written.[15] Some are dreadful: "I swear by the music of the expanding universe and by the eloquence of the good in all of us that I will excite the sick and the well by the severity of my kindness to a wholeness of purpose."[16] Others are witty: "I swear by Humana and . . . health maintenance organizations . . . making them my witnesses, that I will fulfill . . . this oath . . . To hold the one who has taught me this business as equal to my corporation president. . . ."[17] Some medical schools ask each student to write a personal oath based on the Hippocratic Oath.[18] Though the vast majority of U.S. medical schools incorporate an oath into ceremonies for students, only one uses a complete translation of the *Oath*; half use an amended or abridged version and the rest use other oaths.[19] Only a dozen medical schools expose students to *Oath* during their medical ethics education.[20]

The *Oath* faces several possible futures. It could continue to be an honored relic for medical school ceremonies. If so, its language will likely be tweaked with each shift in cultural values to make it work for students who encounter it for the first time and are put off by its anachronistic ideas. It could be quietly dissected in the anatomy labs of scholars of medical history. It could serve as a respected template upon which new statements of medical professionalism are devised. However, if it is a literary classic, its original text can still speak to us if we can learn how to read aright. The *Oath* addresses the perennial issues for medical ethics. I believe that it speaks to us still.

THE *OATH* AS A MEDICAL GRAND ROUNDS

Physicians are storytellers. The most honored teaching method is Grand Rounds—where a skilled physician listens to a story like presentation of a clinical problem and then demonstrates his or her skill at discerning the patient's problem.[21] Today such stories go like this:

> This sixty-five-year-old woman presented to the emergency room with chest pain and heaviness in her arm that began fifteen minutes after eating sushi. She has no fish allergies and does not smoke.

And so it goes: clues and diversions, context and possibilities. The signs and symptoms that are absent are as noteworthy as those that are present. Details are sought. A story emerges like a latent image on film. The coherence and plausibility of this story yield the insight, foresight, and advice that medicine calls *diagnosis*, *prognosis*, and *prescription*. Despite the advent of large-scale research trials, most medical journals still contain case stories in every issue. Medical school tests and specialty board examinations present series of case vignettes for analysis.

It is easy to hear similarities between the narrative case presentations of today and those of Greece. Consider this ancient case report.

> Hippocomus, son of Palamedes in Larissa, eleven years old, was struck on the forehead above the right eye by a horse. The bone did not seem sound and a little blood spurted out of it. He was trephined extensively. And he was cured, despite this condition of the bone, which before was readily festering. [. . .] On the twentieth day, a swelling began by the ear. [. . .] He became fevered.[22]

Greek case records resemble mythic stories. Like the preceding example, many are personalized with names, family names, and places. Even when a personal story is not given, the humanity of the patient is still present. Consider, for example, this ancient trauma surgeon's account of how to assess a person with a head wound.

The first thing to look for in the wounded man is whereabouts in the head the wound is. [. . .] And you should also ask the wounded man how he suffered the injury, and of what kind it is. [. . .] If the bone is not visible, [. . .] it is far more necessary than when the bone is bare to make the interrogation as to the origin and nature of the wound. [. . .] You should first try to distinguish by the patient's report whether the skull has or has not suffered in these ways.[23]

Modern medicine is often criticized for letting technology and an emphasis on objective data depersonalize the physician–patient relationship.

Depersonalization may not be new to medicine. Consider the tone of a typical entry from an Egyptian medical text of 2500 BCE, which describes the assessment of a head wound that is similar to the wound described in the preceding Greek excerpt.

[Title:] Instructions concerning a wound in his head penetrating to the bone of his skull.

[Examination:] If thou examinest a man having a wound in his head, penetrating to bone of his skull, (but) not having a gash, thou shouldst palpate his wound (or, thou shouldst lay thy hand upon it); shouldst thou find his skull uninjured, not having a perforation; a split, or a smash in it.

[Treatment:] Thou shouldst bind it with fresh meat the first day (and) treat afterward with grease, honey (and) lint every day until he recovers.[24]

The personal nature of the Greek case records bespeaks of physicians who willingly engaged in relationships as they went about their technical work.

There is an affinity between Greek medical stories and the dramas of the same culture. Listen to the barely concealed clinical story as Sophocles depicts these citizens presenting the woes afflicting their city to its king, who takes on the role of a secular healer:

CITIZENS: Thebes is dying. A blight on the fresh crops and the rich pastures, cattle sicken and die, and the women die in labor, children stillborn, and the plague, the fiery god of fever hurls down on the city his lightening slashing through us. [. . .] Death luxuriates in the raw wailing miseries of Thebes. [. . .] Thebes, city of death, one long cortege and the suffering rises, wails for mercy rise and the wild hymn for the Healer [Apollo] blazes out.

KING: After a painful search, I have found one cure. You pray to the gods? Let
me grant your prayers. Come, listen to me [. . .] you'll find relief and lift your
head from the depths.[25]

What can Greek plays like Sophocles' *Oedipus the King* add to our understanding of the *Oath*? The tragedies of ancient Greece spoke of and to the Grecian
moral culture at the time when the *Oath* was written.[26] Fifteen thousand people
crowded into the ancient amphitheaters to hear Sophocles, Euripides, and
Aeschylus examine the ethics of relationships, duties, taboos, virtues, weak-
nesses, pride and remorse, good intentions and tragic choices. The Greeks
awarded these dramatists their highest honors. The government valued the
scripts so highly that it legally certified the accuracy of copies.[27] These works
illuminate the moral culture from which the *Oath* originated. They are another tool, along with Greek cultural anthropology and ancient Greek medical treatises, to help us understand its meaning.

If physicians wrote the *Oath*, it may be beneficial to try to listen to *Oath* as a
kind of a case presentation. If so, we should listen to the *Oath* as a coherent whole
rather than as a list of aphorisms. We should listen as one listens to a patient
from another culture, trying to understand how it speaks from the values and
practices of the medical and civic culture from which it came. Many ancient
Greek case records go like this: identify the patient, describe the symptoms, and
make a prognosis for the outcome. The *Oath* has a similar structure:[28]

The physician comes from this heroic family.
A physician acts this way, not that way.
If the physician acts this way, this is what can be hoped for.

In that the *Oath* is about medical ethics, this organization implies a certain
view of medical ethics.

Who are physicians and what is the source of medical professionalism?
To what are physicians committed?
In what way are physicians accountable?

This framework for approaching the moral structure for medical ethics is unfortunately ignored, as most scholarly attention has focused on the ethical

message of specific passages. This framework outlines the fundamental elements of any definition of medical ethics, no matter how different from the *Oath*'s or ours.

THE *OATH*'S MESSAGE FOR TODAY

Ultimately, many readers will want to grapple with what the *Oath* might say to the medical ethics of our time. This is a difficult endeavor that should begin by making a distinction between two ways that the *Oath*'s words may be taken as speaking to contemporary medical ethics.

First, we may find that the *Oath* said something to the medical ethics of its day that still has value for our time. To justify such a finding, it must be demonstrated that the terms, principles, issues, and context that the *Oath* addressed in its time sufficiently resemble those in ours to support applying its words to similar issues today. For example, a passage describes the duty to fully share medical information with one's colleagues and students. Today, as in ancient Greece, physicians and their colleagues and students are engaged in a morally comparable act of creating and transmitting medical knowledge. Today, as in ancient Greece, the purpose of this sharing of information is to sustain the profession and add to medical knowledge. Thus, this moral obligation can be brought forward with little difficulty. In looking at how the Greek physicians spoke of and fulfilled this obligation, we may even learn something of value for our time.

Second, we may choose to accept parts of the *Oath* as speaking to contemporary issues without establishing a historical continuity between its message in its time and the parallel issue in our time. For example, many people see the *Oath*'s disavowal of giving a deadly drug as applicable to the modern debate about physician participation in capital punishment. This is a counterfeit historical foundation in that there is no evidence to support the idea that this passage envisioned or addressed physician participation in executions in ancient Greece. It entails projecting contemporary values and issues back onto ancient Greece and then hearing a historical ratification of those values and issues echoing back to us. The *Oath* has been used in this manner in the debates about medical euthanasia and abortion as well. Conscripting passages of the *Oath* into modern debates in medical ethics in this manner distracts us from recognizing other important ideas for medical ethics that lie in less-attended passages of the *Oath*.

Notwithstanding these difficulties in understanding the *Oath's* message for our time, simply saying that its relevance can't be determined will neither deter nor guide those inclined to attempt this task. Accordingly, most chapters herein close with a speculation on how the *Oath's* passages might be brought forward to the medical ethics of our time. In these closings, I will present cases from my medical career to reflect on how well the cases described by ancient physicians, or the terms and principles described by the *Oath*, resemble or differ from modern counterparts.

Problem-solving by comparing cases, *casuistry*, is one way to try to understand the *Oath's* implications for the medical ethics problems of our time. Casuistry has a long history in philosophy, theology, ethics, and medicine.[29] In medicine, physicians often approach a medical or ethical problem by comparing one case with another. Is this person's disease more like a classic case of pneumonia or a typical case of lung cancer? How is this case of discontinuing life support similar to, or different from, that case of euthanasia? The similarities and differences between cases illuminate significant facts and values and can clarify a diagnosis or help us decide whether the solution to one case applies to the other. Casuistry is a difficult art. Superficially similar cases can differ by morally significant "details." For example, a person with incurable cancer may have a right to refuse life-sustaining treatments, though some believe that feeding by means of a tube into the stomach is a form of care and not a medical treatment at all. The "values" at the center of a debate change over time, notwithstanding any similarity of the technical matter that is being discussed. In our time, the debate about medical abortion centers on the moral status of the fetus relative to a woman's right to control her reproductive life. The *Oath* condemns a physician's use of an abortive pessary, but it is not clear that this conclusion is based on the moral status of a fetus. If the *Oath* does not speak in terms of fetal killing, in what sense is its moral conclusion relevant to our debate about abortion?

Regardless of the extent to which the *Oath* speaks to the pressing issues of our time, its evaluation of the medical ethics of its time is profound and thought provoking. Its pedigree, even if somewhat obscure, can be traced back to the beginning of European scientific medicine. Anyone who reads this text with the goal of thoughtfully accepting, adapting, or rejecting its view of the ethics of medicine will be better equipped to address the crisis of trust facing the medicine of our time. For all these reasons, it deserves a careful reading.

NOTES

1. Lyons JP. The American medical doctor in the current milieu: a matter of trust. Perspectives in Biol Med 1994;37:442–59. Anonymous.

2. Wolfson DB. How to improve trust in health plans. Health Aff 1999;18:269 and Goldberg RK. Regaining public trust. Health Aff 1998;17:138–41.

3. Nutton V. "Hippocratic Morality and Modern Medicine," in Flashar and Jouanna, 31–63.

4. Sealey 95–100.

5. The *Oath* resembles Athenian oratory in using polarities; e.g., slaves and gods, promises and actions, teachers and students, age and youth, past and future. Wills 56–62.

6. Carrick 85–86, 99–100 and Nittis S. The authorship and probable date of the Hippocratic Oath. Bull Hist Med 1940;8:1012–21. Jouanna also accepts early fourth or late fifth century BCE as the date of authorship (Jouanna 401–2).

7. Pellegrino Ed, Pellegrino AA. Humanism and ethics in Roman medicine: Translation and commentary on a text of Scribonius Largus. Lit Med 1988;7:22–38 and Hamilton JS. Scribonius Largus on the medical profession. Bull Hist Med 1986;60:209–16.

8. Nutton V. What's in an oath? J R Coll Phys Lond 1995;29:518–24.

9. Galvao-Sobrinho CR. Hippocratic ideals, medical ethics, and the practice of medicine in the early Middle Ages: The legacy of the Hippocratic Oath. J Hist Med Allied Sci 1996:51:438–55 and Temkin 182–3.

10. See Chapters 4 and 8.

11. Smith DC. The Hippocratic Oath and modern medicine. J Hist Med Allied Sci 1996;51:484–500; Nutton VJ. What's in an oath? J R Coll Physicians Lond 1995;29:518–24.

12. Jones 1924, 23–5. Carrick 181 says this version is third century CE.

13. Temkin 182–3.

14. Pies RW. The "deep structure" of clinical medicine and prescribing privileges for psychologists. J Clin Psychiatry 1991;52:4–8.

15. Declaration of Geneva of the World Medical Association (adopted 1948, amended 1966 and 1983). See also Jewitt DA. Another oath for doctors of medicine

(as written by Howard Brody). N Engl J Med 1975:726; Crawshaw R. A physician's oath for self-insight. Ann Int Med 1979;91:648; Moles AA. A new medical oath. New Engl J Med 307:761; Robin ED. The Hippocratic Oath updated. BMJ 1994;309:96; Andrews BF. Revising the ethics of Hippocrates in the sesquicentennial of Sir William Osler. Kansas Med J 1999;97:431–2; and Manuel BM. A contemporary physician's oath. N Engl J Med 1988;318:521–2.

16. Philipp R, Hart D. An ethical code for everybody in health care: Hippocratic Oath translated into poetry. BMJ 1998;316(7142):1460.

17. Schiedermayer DL. The Hippocratic Oath—Corporate version. New Engl J Med 1986;314:62.

18. Cohn F. Lie D. Mediating the gap between the white coat ceremony and the ethics and professionalism curriculum. Academic Medicine 2002;77:1168.

19. Orr RD, Pang N, Pellegrino ED, Siegler M. Use of the Hippocratic Oath: A review of twentieth century practice and a content analysis of oaths administered in medical school in the US and Canada in 1993. J Clin Ethics 1997;8:374–85.

20. Dubois JM, Burkemper H. Ethics education in US medical schools: A study of syllabi. Acad Med 2002;77432–37.

21. Hunter.

22. *Epidemics 5:16.*

23. *On Wounds of the Head X.*

24. The Egyptian Orthopedic Association maintains a comprehensive website on this papyrus at www.eoa.org.eg/edwintxt.htm#1. See also Wilkins RH. *The Edwin Smith Surgical Papyrus.* Neurosurgery 1964:240–4.

25. Sophocles (1984), Oedipus lines: 30–7, 211–4, 80, 245–7. (See Knox's introduction to Sophocles [1984] 142.) Though Sophocles is known today for his accomplishments in theater and war, Athens gave him an extraordinary hero's funeral because he was the official host when the Asclepian cult was introduced to that *polis* (Knox, notes in Sophocles [1984] 257).

26. For discussions of the use of Greek tragedies in understanding Greek culture, see Nussbaum 1–22, Pearson 8–33, and Patterson 108–9.

27. Casson 26–30.

28. This conceptual parsing is not the same as a grammatical parsing. Von Staden says that there is no clear sentence or paragraph structure in the text that we possess (von Staden H. "'In a pure and holy way:'" Personal and professional conduct in the Hippocratic Oath," J Hist Med Allied Sciences 1996;51:406–8). Some conceptually break the *Oath* down differently. Most commonly, the passage: "I swear by Apollo the Physician . . . to bring the following oath to fulfillment, in accordance with my power and my judgment;" is read as an invocation. In this view, everything that follows is a vow until the entreaty, "If I render this oath fulfilled, and if I do not blur and con-

found it may it be to me to enjoy the benefits . . . If, however, I transgress and perjure myself, the opposite of these."

For reasons that I explain in the introductions to Part I, it is possible to parsing the invocation continuously with the ensuing two passages as defining the lineage of the medical profession. The ensuing promises pertain to the practice of medicine. The closing entreaty remains the same. This parsing reveals an underappreciated strength in how the *Oath's* defines the medicine as a professional lineage.

29. Jonsen and Toulmin 304–22.

I

PHYSICIAN, WHO ARE YOU?

I SWEAR BY APOLLO THE PHYSICIAN AND BY ASCLEPIUS AND
BY HEALTH [HYGIEIA] AND PANACEA AND BY ALL THE GODS AS
WELL AS GODDESSES, MAKING THEM JUDGES [WITNESSES], TO
BRING THE FOLLOWING OATH *AND WRITTEN COVENANT* TO
FULFILLMENT, IN ACCORDANCE WITH MY POWER AND MY
JUDGMENT;
    TO REGARD HIM WHO HAS TAUGHT ME THIS *TECHNÉ*[1] AS
EQUAL TO MY PARENTS, AND TO SHARE, IN PARTNERSHIP, MY
LIVELIHOOD WITH HIM
    AND TO GIVE HIM A SHARE WHEN HE IS IN NEED OF
NECESSITIES, AND TO JUDGE THE OFFSPRING [COMING] FROM
HIM EQUAL TO [MY] MALE SIBLINGS, AND TO TEACH THEM THIS
TECHNÉ, SHOULD THEY DESIRE TO LEARN [IT], WITHOUT FEE
AND WRITTEN COVENANT, AND TO GIVE A SHARE BOTH OF RULES
AND OF LECTURES, AND OF ALL THE REST OF LEARNING, TO MY
SONS AND TO THE [SONS] OF HIM WHO HAS TAUGHT ME AND TO
THE PUPILS WHO HAVE *BOTH MADE A WRITTEN CONTRACT AND
SWORN* BY A MEDICAL CONVENTION BUT BY NO OTHER.

The physician who practiced natural science was a newcomer to ancient
Greece. He arrived as an alternative to Asclepian healers who relied on divination and dreams and who practiced in lavish temples inscribed with testimonials to their miraculous cures.[2] The *Oath*'s opening passages do more than call

upon the gods to witness a physician's swearing to be a moral physician. These words introduce the new arrival, proclaim the lineage of medicine, and tell of the physician's commitments to his teachers and to the future of medicine by contributing to the learning of his colleagues and students. By speaking of teachers and learners, the *Oath* presages the modern French and Latin derived words for healers: *doctors* (a word denoting a teacher) and *physicians* (a word denoting a person who studies medical or natural science).

These opening passages also contain a vow to honor a written contract describing the working and financial arrangements for a medical apprenticeship.[3] Would-be physicians arranged to work as apprentices to senior physicians. As far as we know, there was no specified length to the apprenticeship, no core curriculum, and no licensure or certification at its completion. The teacher and apprentice split the revenues from their work.[4] The *Oath* notes that some students, except those who were the sons of physicians, paid tuition to a teacher in addition to working as apprentices. It is possible that other oaths, lost to history, may have specified other financial relationships. The references to this contract are shown in *italics* in the excerpt above. They are conceptually distinct from the passages that address the ethics of the profession as healers and will not be addressed further.

NOTES

1. *Techné* is defined in Chapter 8.
2. Aleshire 52–72.
3. Nittis S. The authorship and probable date of the Hippocratic Oath. Bull Hist Med 1940;8:1012–21. Drabkin IE. Medical Education in ancient Greece and Rome. J Med Ed 1957;32:286–395. Jouanna 47–48, 128–9.
4. Jouanna 370–2.

2

CREATORS

I SWEAR BY APOLLO THE PHYSICIAN AND BY ASCLEPIUS AND
BY HEALTH [HYGIEIA] AND PANACEA AND BY ALL THE GODS AS
WELL AS GODDESSES, MAKING THEM JUDGES [WITNESSES],
TO BRING THE FOLLOWING OATH ... TO FULFILLMENT, IN
ACCORDANCE WITH MY POWER AND MY JUDGMENT. . . .

In ancient Greece, new arrivals called out their ancestry and homeland. Here is how the playwright Euripides has Amphitryon introduce himself:

> Is there a man living who has not heard of me—Amphitryon of Argos, whose bed welcomed Zeus? Son of Alcaeus, grandson of Perseus; and father of Heracles. I have lived here in Thebes ever since the crop of Sown Men sprang full-grown out of the earth. . . .[1]

The opening passage of the *Oath* deftly combines the convention of swearing by a god with proclaiming the physician's lineage.[2] This lineage starts with Apollo, proceeds to his son Asclepius, and includes Asclepius's divine daughters Panacea and Hygieia. Asclepius's human sons were heroic physicians themselves, and legend names one as an ancestor of Hippocrates. In the next chapter, we shall see how the *Oath* has each physician become part of this lineage. A person who claimed such a noble lineage was destined to play an important role in society and merited a respectful hearing.

WHY SWEAR BY APOLLO?

Why did the ancient physicians not swear by the most powerful god, Zeus? After all, Greek medicine was weak; diseases and injuries were often intractable; and remedies were often ineffective. Nearly two-thirds of the patients described in the ancient Greek medical treatises died under the physician's care. Why swear by Apollo and not by Zeus? Our culture does not prepare us to hear the significance of the proclamation "I swear by Apollo." Epigrams such as "Apollo is the god of poetry, healing, prophesy, and reason" only hint at the meanings embedded in the stories that we call myths.

Apollo was passionate about humans.[3] He fell in love with the human woman Coronis and they made love. He went off and left a white crow to watch over her in his absence. The crow came to Apollo and told him that Coronis had fallen in love with another; his rage blackened the crow. He told his sister, Artemis, to shoot Coronis with an arrow. The dying Coronis whispered that she was carrying his son. Grief stricken, "Apollo the Physician" plied his medical skill in vain. As the pyre's flames consumed her body, Apollo reached into her and pulled forth Asclepius. Apollo asked the wise centaur, Chiron, to raise and instruct him. Chiron taught Asclepius medicine and, like other humans with a divine parent, Asclepius excelled.[4]

Asclepius married Epione, a noted healer in her own right. She was a daughter of Heracles, and their children signify the diverse branches of health and healing. Two daughters are mentioned in the *Oath*: Hygieia (goddess of health or preventive health care) and Panacea (All-Heal, goddess of remedies). There were three other divine offspring: Iaso (goddess of medicine, from which the word *iatros*, meaning "physician," comes), Aigle (radiance), and a deified son, Telesphorus (god of convalescence). Asclepius and Epione also had two human sons, Machaon and Podalirius. Homer names Asclepius as a historical lord who sent his sons Podalirius and Machaon, both skilled healers, to lead troops in the Trojan War.[5] Machaon was killed as part of the force that entered Troy in the Wooden Horse.[6] Podalirius survived the war and traveled south to settle on the Ionian coast of the Mediterranean Sea, an area that is now part of Turkey. His descendents sailed to the nearby island of Cos, which is still part of Greece. Hippocrates came from a family of healers that legend says is descended from Podalirius and thus from Asclepius.[7]

Asclepius died because he transgressed as a physician. Athene had given him two vials of blood from the right arm of the Medusa, which he used to bring Capaneus, Glaucus, Hippolytus, and Tyndareus to life from death. The Greek poet Pindar tells the story this way:

> Still, even wisdom yields to hope of profit. And gold induced no less than he [Asclepius] to try to resurrect a man whom death already had imprisoned. . . . We must seek from deity the things that fit our mortal hearts, keeping our condition and our destiny in mind. My vital being, do not seek immortal life; exhaust, instead, all possibility.[8]

Hades noticed the missing dead and complained to Zeus about the physician's threat to his domain. Apollo, through Euripides, tells what happens next:

> Zeus killed my son, Asclepius, and drove the bolt of the hot lightening through his chest. I, in my anger for this, killed the Cyclopes, smith of Zeus's fire, for which my father [Zeus] made me serve a mortal man, in penance for my misdoings. I came to this country, tended the oxen of this house and friend, Admetus, son of Pheres.[9]

Eventually, Zeus's rage abated and he acknowledged Asclepius' gift of medicine by deifying him and placing his star in the sky.[10] Apollo's contest with death continued for several more myth cycles.[11]

The stories of Asclepius offer clues to why the ancient physicians did not swear by Ares, the god of war. Modern medicine freely analogizes medicine to war and has declared wars on cancer, AIDS, drug abuse, and heart disease.[12] Rescue sorties into the land of the dead figure prominently in many Greek myths. Greek physicians did not see themselves as waging a war against disease. Instead, they sought to gently turn the body toward its natural health by working with innate forces to restore a harmonious balance. Throughout the ancient medical literature there is advice like, "The body's nature is the physician in disease,"[13] or, "The progress of a disease should be guided, where guidance is needed, so that it develops in its most favorable manner according to its natural tendency."[14] The name "Asclepius" means "unceasingly gentle." His healing wife's name, Epione, means "soothing." These were not warrior healers.

Apollo merits being invoked by the *Oath* for more reasons than simply being known as "Physician" and fathering Asclepius. He was also the god of reason and the god of prophecy and of the Oracle at Delphi, where an active temple existed before and during the time of the *Oath*. Greeks pioneered the study of rational cause and effect. With reason, Greek physicians forged a natural science of medicine by attributing symptoms to natural, rather than divine, causes.[15] As an ancient Greek medical text, *Epidemics II*, says, "One must approach the cause, and of the cause, the source."[16] The Greek physicians took the logic of natural "causes and effects" a remarkable step further. If reasoning by cause and effect could explain how the past led to a present illness, it could also be used to infer a future condition from a present one. Physicians could not prophesy like the Delphic Oracle but they did take pride in their prognostic ability.

Ancient Greek medical texts devote many pages to rules for making prognoses—the medical prophecies and for untangling the conundrums of why one person with a disease dies while another, similarly afflicted person, lives. These are from *Aphorisms*.

> If a patient suffering from fever, with no swelling in the throat, be suddenly seized with suffocation, it is a deadly symptom.[17]

> Those who are attacked by tetanus either die in four days, or if they survive these, recover.[18]

It takes a great deal of experience to make such prognostic inferences. Signs are hard to read. Predictions are often unwelcome. Excessive pride in one's skill as a diagnostician or as a healer can lead to mistakes. Misplaced confidence in one's prognoses causes regrettable moments in medicine, as when a person who is given a clean bill of health is discovered to be ill or a person who is deemed mortally ill goes on to recover. The same was true in Greece; one of the ancient *Aphorisms* cautions: "In the case of acute diseases, to predict either death or recovery is not quite safe."[19]

Whom, then, would physicians claim as their divine forebear? Ares, god of war, does not embody the tender spirit of this new profession. Zeus, though powerful, slew Asclepius and enslaved his father, Apollo. The Greek physicians grounded their profession and medicine's future on Apollo's arts of healing, reason, and prognostication. Apollo—the Physician—god of poetry, healing, prophecy, and reason founded the house of medicine. Socrates describes the aptness of Apollo's association with medicine this way, "Is not Apollo the purifier, and the washer, and the absolver from all impurities? . . . Then, in reference to his ablutions and absolutions, as being the physician who orders them, he may be rightly called Apolouon (purifier); or in respect of his powers of divination, and his truth and sincerity, which is the same as truth, he may be most fitly called Aplos, from *aplous* (sincere)."[20]

Though the *Oath* only names gods, the titan Prometheus, whose name means "forethought," deserves mention. He is most often remembered for being condemned by Zeus for giving humans the gift of fire, and with it, heat, cooking, smelting, and scores of other inventions. Fire is emblematic of the gift of the spirit of invention, imagination, and foresight that humans apply to their needs. As Aeschylus imagines him, here is what Prometheus claims to have done for humans:

> They had eyes but no eyes to see and ears but heard not. . . . They knew not how to build brick houses to face the sun, nor work in wood. They lived beneath the earth like swarming ants in sunless caves . . . until it was I that showed to them stars' risings, . . . and numbering as well, preeminent of subtle devices, and letter combinations that hold all in memory. . . . I was the first to yoke beast to be slave to the traces . . . and carriages that wander on the sea, the ship sail-winged. . . .
>
> Greatest was this: when one of mankind was sick, there was no defense for him—neither healing food nor drink nor unguent; for lack of drugs they wasted until I showed them blendings of mild simples with which they drive away all kinds of sickness.
>
> The many ways of prophesying I charted. . . .
>
> In one short sentence understand it all: every art of mankind comes from Prometheus.[21]

Prometheus gave humans the inventiveness that drives the art and science of medicine. Yet, he limited this gift of forethought in a way that has momentous importance to medicine. Aeschylus quotes Prometheus:

> PROMETHEUS: I stopped mortals from foreseeing doom.
> CHORUS: What cure did you discover for that sickness?
> PROMETHEUS: I sowed in them blind hopes.[22]

Physicians and patients cannot foresee the time and manner of a person's death. As death nears, hope for recovery or cure will skew each party's judgment about the prognosis or the efficacy of the treatment. The physician's prognostication resembles prophecy but human foresight is no equal of divine prescience.

SECULAR AND SACRED MEDICINE IN CLASSIC GREECE

The ancient Greek medical treatises reject divine explanations for disease, as well as healing prayers and blessings. Consider this excerpt from an essay on epilepsy, then called "the sacred disease":

> I do not believe that the "Sacred Disease" is any more divine or sacred than any other disease. . . . It is my opinion that those who first called this disease "sacred" were the sort of people we now call witch doctors, faith healers, quacks and charlatans. These are exactly the people who pretend to be very pious and be particularly wise. By invoking a divine element they were able to screen their own failure to give suitable treatment and so called this a "sacred" malady to conceal their ignorance of its nature. . . . I believe that this disease is not in the least more divine than any other but has the same nature as other diseases and a similar cause. Moreover, it can be cured no less than other diseases so long as it has not become inveterate and too powerful for the drugs which are given. . . . [A] man with the knowledge of how to produce [a treatment] . . . would not need to resort to purifications and magic spells.[23]

This kind of secular and natural understanding of disease separated physicians from gods and priests and made a natural science of medicine possible.

A clinical application of this separation is vividly illustrated in another ancient medical text, *Airs, Waters, Places*, which describes the medical investigation of an area where the gods are blamed for the impotence of wealthy men. The author notes that if the condition had a divine origin, it should afflict all classes equally, or perhaps even spare the rich, who could afford the most lavish sacrifices to please the gods. "But the truth is . . . these affections are neither more nor less divine than any others and all and each are natural."[24] The impotence, he says, is caused by the fact that only the rich can afford to experience the trauma, fatigue, and arthritis caused by horseback riding.

The contrast between secular physicians and the Asclepian healers can be seen from testimonial inscriptions of treatment at Asclepian temples:[25]

A man came as a supplicant to the god. He was so blind that of one of his eyes he had only the eyelids left—within them was nothing, but they were entirely empty. Some of those in the Temple laughed at his silliness to think that he could recover his sight when one of his eyes had not even a trace of the ball. . . . As he slept, a vision appeared to him. It seemed to him that the god prepared some drug, then opening his eyelids poured it into them. When day came, he departed with the sight of both eyes restored.[26]

The transition from divine to scientific healing was neither instantaneous nor complete.[27] Though faith in religious healing was beginning to decline by the fifth century BCE, a wise physician deferred to conventional piety and the powerful temple healers.[28] As one physician put it, "prayer indeed is good, but while calling on the gods a man should lend himself a hand."[29] The separation played out in the competition for business between physicians and healer-priests. Greek medicine was often ineffective; physician's critiques of sacred healing (like the passage quoted above) noted that divine healers were arbitrary and often ineffective. The author of *Prorrhetic II* wryly distinguished between those who prophesied that a healthy person would become lame and those who made a prognosis of lameness from their assessment of an illness: "those who make predictions about lameness and other conditions of that kind make their predictions, if they are sensible, only after the disease has become fixed . . . rather than before."[30] The broader society honored both secular and sacred healers, even on Cos, the birthplace of Hippocrates,[31] even as Sophocles wrote this biting comment on faith healers, "tis not a skillful leech who mumbles charms over ills that need the knife."[32] Even today, healing maintains a sense of the divine about it.

Just as people today simultaneously see physicians while they pray and take naturopathic preparations, there was a lot of blended medicine in ancient Greece. Some patients did not distinguish the natural medicine of prognostication from healing based on divination.[33] Some hedged their bets using both secular and divine healers. Scholars going back to Socrates have noted that ancient medical therapies overlapped with purifying rituals of the ill.[34] Consider this treatment for pleurisy: "On the fourth day give baths, on the fifth and sixth days anoint with olive oil, and on the seventh day wash."[35] The ancient Greek physicians carved out a niche for their science but in no way established hegemony over the field of healing.

CHRISTIANS AND SWEARING BY APOLLO

The *Oath*'s invocation of Apollo has posed a problem for religious persons for at least 1,700 years.[36] Several solutions have been proposed.

- Some accept the *Oath* as written, taking its Apollonian reference simply as a historical signature that can be freely excised and replaced with other deities.[37] An eleventh century version for Christians began, "Blessed be God the Father of our Lord Jesus Christ, who is blessed for ever and ever; I lie not."[38]
- Some reconstruct the entire *Oath* to conform to a Christian position.[39] As one author puts it, "To reform medicine, we must Christianize the Hippocratic Oath."[40] The National Catholic Bioethics Center rewrites the prologue this way, "I swear in the presence of the Almighty and before my family, my teachers and my peers."[41] The Center goes on to rewrite the passages on abortion and poison and calls the transformed document "The 1995 Restatement of the Oath of Hippocrates, circa 400 B.C."
- Some Christian writers argue that the *Oath* is a pre-Christian text that is fundamentally compatible with the ensuing Christian ethics. In this view, the moral vision of the *Oath* may be accepted, much like Thomas Aquinas fitted many of Aristotle's ideas into Catholic theology.[42]

Each of these solutions is still very much a part of the current reception of the *Oath*.

Regardless of the demise of the religion of the Olympian gods, modern readers do well to reflect on the message embedded in the Apollonian opening. It is not a simple invocation of some god, any god, to witness the vow to be a good physician. The *Oath* names Apollo, Asclepius, Hygieia, and Panacea for a reason. Each name intones a moral chord that is then linked to another in myths to form moral songs. The words "I swear by Apollo . . ." reverberate with a cosmology that sings of the origins, purposes, and limits of medicine. Apollo's valiant effort to save his beloved Coronis, and how this effort leads to dedicating Asclepius to healing, speaks of how the passion to heal is grounded on love and grief. Apollo's failure to save the human Coronis who was struck down by a god, as well as the story of the punishment of Asclepius for resurrecting the dead teach that medicine must accept human mortality as the proper moral boundary for its work. The gentleness that suffuses the very names of Asclepius and Epione speaks of a healing art that is not at war with disease or the body but that seeks to work with the body to turn it to health. Such gentleness is a recurring theme in many of the ancient medical works.[43] Finally, these opening lines do not leave the physician as a mere spectator in this moral drama. Asclepius is a descendent of Apollo, and the physician joins them as a descendent in the *Oath*'s next passage.

NOTES

1. Euripides, *Heracles* 1–4. The lineage going back to a divine progenitor may be an example of a Greek institution called a *phratry*, roughly "brotherhood." These were important multifamilial and geographically dispersed organizations. It is tempting to consider whether physicians constituted a *phratry*. They did place themselves in the lineage of Apollo by way of Asclepius, Podalirius, and Hippocrates. It is unusual, however, to affirm divine female ancestry, though Panacea and Hygieia were sisters of Podalirius and not interposed in the patrilineal descent from Apollo. The *Oath* is sworn by adults, whereas entry to a *phratry* generally occurred during infancy (Pomeroy 1988, 36, 74–82).

2. Sealy (95–100) notes that a Homeric oath invocation need not simply call upon a god as a witness, it can swear by a thing of awe such as a marriage bed, a sword, or a home.

3. Graves (1964) is used as the reference for myths. There are variant tellings of myths. Readers who are interested in these should consult specialized references.

4. Edelstein and Edelstein (1945) is a compendium of the classic quotations referring to Asclepius.

5. Homer (eighth century BCE) says that Asclepius was a lord within the city of King Eurytus. He speaks of this when he details the massing of the Greek forces against Troy: "Now I can only tell the lords of the ships, the ships in all their numbers! . . . Oechalia, Eurytus' city: the two sons of Asclepius led their units now, both skilled healers, Podalirius and Machaon. In their command sailed forty curved black ships," (*Iliad*, II: 582–3, 831–6). Troy fell in about 1200 BCE.

6. Jouanna 420, n 22.

7. The Apollonian-Asclepian ancestry of Hippocrates causes a fair amount of confusion. Some people mistakenly believe that the *Oath* is a priestly oath or that the Hippocratic School was a temple-based healing cult. Asclepian physicians were priestly healers who claimed to be descendents of Asclepius (Aleshire). They were affiliated with temples to Asclepius and they healed by prayer, sacrifice, divination, and naturo-

pathic cures. By virtue of his descent through Podalirius, Hippocrates was an Asclepian physician and would have had the privilege to practice in the temples (Joanna 34–35, 45–50). The *Oath*, however, specifically opens the profession to the unrelated pupils who have both made a written contract and "sworn by a medical convention." In this sense, the *Oath* departs from the familial lineage claimed by Asclepian physicians; thus it is corrupt to use *Asclepian* to refer to any physician.

   8. Pindar. *Pythian Odes* 3–63.

   9. Euripides. *Alcestis* 3–8.

   10. Asclepius is a star. A constellation memorializes his teacher, Chiron.

   11. Admetus was the father of Hippolytus, one of the people whom Asclepius brought back from the dead. Later, Apollo tricked the Fates into agreeing to postpone his friend Admetus' death with the condition that someone would volunteer to die for him at his fated hour. His wife, Alcestis, agreed to die in his stead. Heracles brought her back from the dead.

   12. Lerner (2001) and Sontag 65–9 discuss war metaphors in medicine.

   13. *Epidemics* 6.5:1. See also Carella 281–3.

   14. *Aphorisms I:21* (translation from Hippocrates 1950).

   15. Jouanna 179–259.

   16. *Epidemics* 2.4:5.

   17. *Aphorisms IV:xxxiv.*

   18. *Aphorisms V:vi.*

   19. *Aphorisms II:19*

   20. *Cratylus* 405b-c.

   21. Aeschylus, *Prometheus Bound*, 448–507.

   22. Aeschylus, *Prometheus Bound*, 250–3.

   23. *The Sacred Disease: 1, 2, 4, 5, 21* (Translation from Hippocrates 1950).

   24. *Airs, Waters, Places: 22.*

   25. Aleshire has a detailed discussion of Asclepian temples.

   26. Edelstein and Edelstein 424–5.

   27. This medical secularism did not, and could not, occur in isolation from comparable trends in the larger society during Greece of the Classical period (Lloyd [1979] 10–58); Jouanna 181–209; Temkin 80–5.

   28. Aleshire 52–72 describes the wealth and aristocratic nature of the temple healers.

   29. *On Regimen IV:LXXXVII.*

   30. *Prorrhetic II:2*

   31. Langhoff 234–5.

   32. Sophocles, *Ajax, 581–2.*

   33. Langhoff 233.

34. Parker 1986–7. Plato quotes Socrates discussing the significance of the association of Apollo with physicians: "In the first place, the purgations and purifications which doctors and diviners use, and their fumigations with drugs magical or medicinal, as well as their washings and lustral sprinklings, have all one and the same object, which is to make a man pure both in body and soul. And is not Apollo the purifier, and the washer, and the absolver from all impurities?"(Plato, *Cratylus 404e–405c*)

35. *Places in Man 17.*

36. Temkin 182–3.

37. "Apollo—or whatever its name is—brings wholeness to mind and us to wholeness, and further in the art of medicine, brings us beyond awareness of wholeness to a divine like overflowing into action. . . ." (Kass 244–5).

38. Jones (1924) 23–25. Carrick says this is third century (181). Temkin takes no position on the date (183).

39. Verhey A. The doctors' oath—and a Christian swearing it. Linacre Quarterly 1984;51:139–58.

40. Finnell V. Reforming Medicine. Chalcedon Rep 2001;(Jan):42–6.

41. Value of Life Committee. "The 1995 restatement of the Oath of Hippocrates, circa 400 BC." National Catholic Center, Boston, MA 02135 [www.ncbcenter.org]

42. See Winslow GR. Christian theology and the Hippocratic Oath. Update (Center for Christian Bioethics of Loma Linda University) 1998;14(1):6–7. (www.llu.edu/llu/bioethics/). Fiorenzo Cardinal Angelini. The meaning of a historical trajectory. www.vatican.va/roman_curia/pontifical_councils/hlthwork/documents/rc_pc_hlthwork_doc_09061997_angelini-art_en.html.

43. "Dexterity [in bandaging] is as follows: . . . what you must take hold gently, to take hold of and not to press tight: when bandaging not to make uneven twists or to apply pressure where you should not; when palpating, wherever you do, not to cause unnecessary pain. (*Diseases I:10*)." In surgery, "practice all the operations, performing them with each hand and with both together—for they are both alike—your object being to attain ability, grace, speed, painlessness, elegance and readiness (*In the Surgery IV*),"or "In cases where the surgery is performed by a single incision, you must make it a quick one; for since the person being cut generally suffers pain, this suffering should last for the least time possible. . . . However, when many incisions are necessary, you must employ a slow surgery, for a surgeon that was fast would make the pain sustained and great, whereas intervals provide a break in its intensity for the patients. (*Physician 5*)" It also extends to demeanor: "Kindnesses to those who are ill. For example, to do in a clean way his food or drink or whatever he sees; softly, what he touches. Things that do not great harm and are easily got, such as a cold drink when it is needed. Manner of entrance, conversation. Position and clothing for the sick person, hair, nails, scents (*Epidemics 6;4:7*)."

3

TEACHERS

... [T]O REGARD HIM WHO HAS TAUGHT ME THIS *TECHNÉ*[1] (ART
AND SCIENCE) AS EQUAL TO MY PARENTS, AND TO SHARE, IN
PARTNERSHIP, MY LIVELIHOOD WITH HIM AND TO GIVE HIM A
SHARE WHEN HE IS IN NEED OF NECESSITIES. ...

This passage extends the lineage, inserts the physician into that family, and
defines the first of two familial obligations of physicians to this house of medicine. The lineage of medicine began with the *Oath's* summoning of Apollo,
Asclepius, Panacea, and Hygieia as witnesses and progenitors of medicine. In
this passage, a physician enters the professional family of physicians by accepting his medical teachers as equal to his parents. Furthermore, the physician
vows to assume filial obligations to the preceding generation of teachers.

The vow to provide for one's teachers in the event of their need resonates
with the expected answer to a question that was publicly asked of aspirants to
Greek public office: "Do you treat your parents well?"[2] In this answer, the
physician proclaims that the filial relationship is profound rather than simply
symbolic. Moreover, by positing the future neediness of one's teachers as en-
tailing a moral obligation, the *Oath* implicitly recognizes that professional
generations pass like the passing of generational authority in families. In families, the infirmity of elders creates two kinds of duties: a duty to care for the

parent and a duty to assume family leadership so that the house continues to flourish. Nothing else is known about how that first obligation was historically fulfilled. The second duty, addressed in the following passage, is discussed in the next chapter. This is, however, an appropriate point to reflect on how Hippocrates' professional descendants have regarded their ancestor.

HIPPOCRATES

Admirers have diligently searched for information about the historical Hippocrates.[3] It is certain that he was an actual person who was born in 460 BCE on the Greek island of Cos. His immediate forebears were prominent healers. Nothing is known of his childhood or medical training, though the latter presumably included a medical apprenticeship in the family. It is said that he married well, though his wife's name is unknown. His two sons and a son-in-law, Polybus, became physicians. After his parents died, he moved to Thessaly on the Greek mainland, possibly leaving the medical center in Cos under the leadership of Polybus. Some say he moved because of a dispute with a competing medical school on a nearby island, Cnidos. Some say that he set fire to its library. Some say that a dream sent him to Thessaly. Some say that he left Cos to broaden his knowledge of medicine or to study the relationship between various environments and health. Academic quarrels, scandal, dreams, whim, and the pursuit of science: professors are nomadic today for the same reasons.

There are no extant records of the life and journeys of Hippocrates and his colleagues. He lived to an old age, reportedly dying in Larissa, a town in Thessaly, in about 375 BCE. Why Larissa? Perhaps he died where he was reputedly practicing. Many of the patients described in case records written during Hippocrates' life lived in the region of Thessaly; some even lived in Larissa. There is no evidence, however, to confirm that Hippocrates himself treated these people or wrote these records. It is possible that the story of his death in Larissa could be the final melding of the history and myth of Hippocrates. Larissa was the home of Coronis, the love of Apollo and mother of Asclepius. Larissa is near Oechalia, the town from which Homer says the historical Asclepius sent his son and Hippocrates' legendary ancestor, Podalirius, to be a physician-commander in the Trojan War.[4] After his death, some revered Hippocrates as a holy man or even as a deity. Ancient forgers created a variety of documents describing his activities.[5] Miracles reportedly occurred at his grave.

The commingling of legend, myth, and hagiography in the biography of Hippocrates attests to the fact that almost nothing is known about him. We know that he enjoyed a reputation as a gifted physician, but not one quote, case record, or medical treatise — not even the *Oath* — is securely attributed to him. We know that he was respected as a natural philosopher and as a participant in the momentous intellectual developments of his time.[6] We know that he or members of his circle articulated a natural science of medicine and distinguished it from a temple-based medicine that understood sickness as the effect of curses or divine disfavor and healing as occurring through divination, prayer, anointment, and sacrifice. It is fair to infer that he was a powerful teacher and author. We know nothing, however, about his personality, habits, or peccadilloes. Reliable sources indicate that he went bald.

HIPPOCRATES IN THE CHRISTIAN WEST

Given such scanty facts, it was Christian Europe's construction of Hippocrates as the ancient Greek physician of record that has so profoundly shaped our view of him and of the stature and the meaning of the *Oath*. For its first three centuries, Christianity existed side by side with the Roman and Greek pantheons, including the deified Asclepius. Eventually, Christians asserted the exclusive supremacy of their God. The cult of the pagan Asclepius was suppressed, while respect for Hippocrates, a consummate human physician, was allowed to endure.[7] During this time, Christian theologians labored to create an acceptable understanding of the science of healing in a universe where God was the understood to be the true healer and death was a part of His plan.[8] As noted in Chapter 1, the *Oath* was rarely mentioned during the first 1,500 years of Christianity. It was also peripheral to the medical ethics of the first Christian millennium, which drew on evolving Christian views on love of people (*philanthropia*), charity, and compassionate empathy (*misericordia*).[9] Eventually, church scholars came to accept an often-modified *Oath* as an exemplary pre-Christian statement of the ethical duties of physicians.[10] Even so, as Dante put it, Hippocrates belonged to the "time of the false Gods of lying fame." Dante wrote of seeing the "supreme Hippocrates whom Nature for her dearest creatures made" among the nobles of the ancient world who "sinned not," in Limbo—the first circle of Hell.[11]

Hippocrates' subsequent rise rests on a transformation of the view of his role in the history of European medical science.[12] In the second century, Galen compiled and discussed the Greek medical treatises. He recast the pathophysiology and treatments of Hippocratic medicine to conform to his own views and bequeathed them to the Middle Ages, when they became the core of medical education.[13] From the sixteenth to the nineteenth centuries, Galen's bequest of a static and iconic classical medical lore was transformed. Thomas Sydenham and René Laennec, for example, recast Hippocrates from being the author of obsolete lore to being the creative force behind the development of an empirical, progressing, and anti-dogmatic science.[14] The nineteenth-century physician-linguist Paul Emile Littré translated the Hippocratic works into French. His translation and commentary, entitled "Complete Works of Hippocrates," is the foundation for modern Hippocratic studies.[15]

Thus, religion and science delivered Hippocrates, "The Father of Medicine," to the twentieth century as the author of record of the method for the natural science of medicine and of the iconic statement of medical ethics. A puzzle remained. How could the *Oath* have articulated a Christian medical ethic centuries before Jesus was born?

In the 1940s, Ludwig Edelstein proposed to resolve this paradox by attributing the *Oath* to philosophers.[16] He concluded that Greek physicians' rules for medical practice were simply conventions for bedside etiquette. When he made that conclusion, the intellectual endeavor that we know as medical ethics, or more specifically, clinical ethics had yet not been created. It is probably not a coincidence that the medical ethics of Edelstein's own time was articulated by Thomas Percival and the American Medical Association (AMA) and was essentially a guild ethic of bedside decorum. In Edelstein's view, Pythagorean philosophers, rather than physicians, created the foundation of medical ethics: "I think that in antiquity, philosophy influenced medicine rather than being influenced by it." In his view, this accounted for the divergence between the ethical norms described in the *Oath* and Greek practice as described in the medical works. For example, the *Oath* disavows surgery even though Greek physicians were aggressive surgeons. He concluded that the *Oath* anticipated and eventually was fulfilled in Christian medical ethics because the Pythagoreans were proto-Christians.[17]

A new religion arose that challenged the very foundations of ancient civilization. Yet, Pythagoreanism seemed to bridge the gulf between heathendom and the new belief. Christianity found itself in agreement with the principles of Pythagorean ethics, its concepts of holiness and purity, justice and forbearance. The Pythagorean god who forbade suicide to men, his creatures, was also the God of the Jews and the Christians.[18]

Today, many medical ethicists uncritically cite Edelstein's conclusion that the *Oath* is of Pythagorean derivation[19] even though most scholars of ancient Greece are at least skeptical of the claim that the *Oath* written by Pythagorean philosophers.[20] Though Edelstein's hypothesis is widely doubted by scholars of ancient medicine, his critics have not advanced an alternative explanation of the *Oath* as a statement of a medical ethics of ancient Greece.

Hippocrates is something like a black hole. Unseen and unknown, his enormous gravitas shapes and spins the galaxy of Western medicine. The constant reinterpretation of ancient Greek medicine and the attribution of that culture's medicine to Hippocrates have secured his name at the center of the medical heavens.

*   *   *

CASE 3.1 When I was a child, an aunt became "very sick." She began to miss the family gatherings. In those not so distant days, the word "cancer" was breathed, rather than spoken aloud. After some months, I was taken to see her in a hospital. It was a good-bye visit where "good-bye" were unspeakable words. She was thin and pale. Her face was the friendly face I knew, but it had a tautness that, years later, I would learn to recognize as a sign of chronic pain. I recall being horrified by her left arm. It was hugely swollen, wrapped in bandages, and propped up on pillows. A soft, bulbous hand protruded from the bandages. "How could a disease do that?" I wondered. Later, I learned that this swelling was caused by the Halsted operation.

My aunt had undergone a radical mastectomy. This operation attempted to cure breast cancer by removing all the sites where a cancer might have silently spread. In addition to the breast, the muscles of the chest, as well as lymph nodes in the chest, armpit and lower neck were removed. Since the lymph ducts could no longer drain fluid from the arm through the nodes, the arm became swollen with edema.

Medical terminology memorializes countless Greek gods, stories, and heroes.[21] There is the Atlas vertebrae, the Delphian node, Faun's beard, hermaphrodite, hymen, and iris. Physicians treat chimerism, Ondine's curse, priapism, Proteus syndrome, sirenomelia and morbus herculeus. They employ aphrodisiacs, atropine, cycloplegics, hygiene, hypnotics, hypnotism, and Minerva jackets while searching for panaceas. A field named for Psyche has named complexes for Cassandra, Diana, Electra, Icarus, Medea, Oedipus, Orestes, Sisyphus, and Ulysses in addition to echolalia, erotomania, narcissism, nymphomania, and satyriasis. There is Promethean genetics and thanatology, the latter term being applied to early ethics committees that dealt largely with the moral dilemmas at the end of life. Only one Greek human was memorialized. Hippocrates earned five eponyms: Hippocratic fingers (pulmonary osteoarthropathy, the bulbous fingertips that signify chronic lung disease), Hippocratic facies (the face of someone who is in shock with impending death), Hippocratic succussion splashes (shaking a patient to hear a sloshing of fluid around the lung), Hippocratic tumors (malignant melanoma of the skin), and Hippocrates' method (fixing an anterior dislocation of shoulder by applying traction with the hands against counter-traction by a foot in the armpit).

Medical eponyms are a slowly disappearing art. Gods' names are no longer used. Today, medical heroes are honored: Parkinson disease, Koch's postulates, the Wangensteen tube, the Salk vaccine, pasteurization, Babinski reflex, the Apgar score of a newborn's health, and the Halsted procedure. Each such star turns in the medical heavens; some to set as time passes and new insights and new constellations rise to take their place.

The rising and setting of honorific eponyms speaks of the temporal nature of generational authority in medicine. Like aging parents, physicians can lose their greatness. Some insights are proven wrong. Some techniques are superseded. Excessive deference to great teachers, like undue deference to a failing parent, can harm the estate and reputation of a family. So it was with the enormous professional deference given to the eminent surgeon Dr. William Halsted (1852–1922).[22]

Dr. Halsted's surgery for breast cancer, the operation that bears his name, was based on an inaccurate theory. An ancient Greek surgeon, with special skill in orthopedics, somewhat unfairly said, "The theorizing practitioners are just the ones who go wrong."[23] Dr. Halsted proposal seemed logical enough: breast cancer cells metastasize like invaders from a beachhead—first to adjoining breast tissue, then to nearby muscles, next to regional lymph nodes, and finally to the rest of the body. He concluded that a surgeon who found breast cancer should immediately remove all of these structures to eradicate the tumor and its spreading seeds. In truth, some breast cancers spread early and widely throughout the body and others do not. Halsted's deforming and disabling procedure was more than what was needed for tumors that had not spread and offered no advantage for those that had. His powerful exposition of the procedure left an indelible mark on generations of physicians.

Dr. Sherwin Nuland, a surgeon who adhered to the Halsted procedure long after data showed it to be unnecessary, explained his loyalty by tracing his lineage to Dr. Halsted. "I was trained by Gustaf Lindskog, who was trained by Samuel Harvey, who was trained by Halsted's first resident, Harvey Cushing."[24] Such filial devotion led surgeons to resist decades of evidence showing no advantage over less aggressive surgery from the extensive, debilitating, and disfiguring Halsted procedure.

Dr. George Crile, Jr. had a notably different familial upbringing. He followed his eminent father into a surgical career. As the younger surgeon's skill advanced, cataracts and glaucoma impaired his father's vision. While they operated together, Dr. Crile corrected his father's surgical missteps and experienced increasing distress over the conflict between loyalty to his father and duty to needlessly endangered patients.[25] Dr. Crile was trained in the Halsted mastectomy and used it exclusively for seventeen years. About 1950, European surgeons were reporting that a simple mastectomy resulted in comparable longevity with less disability. Dr. Crile's experience with his failing father was a formative lesson: he became an ardent American critic of the radical mastectomy and withstood the fire of his colleagues. Halsted's intensely loyal professional sons lambasted the "dour wizards" of statistics who rejected "the art of medicine."[26] The Halsted mastectomy was eventually abandoned, but misplaced filial devotion kept it in practice long enough to needlessly compound my aunt's suffering in the mid-1960s.

Experiences like these have led to calls for "evidence-based medicine."[27] This oddly self-evident term refers to looking to research to evaluate the evidence that a given therapy will benefit a particular patient. Thus a therapy must not only be theoretically sound or beneficial in the hands and eyes of its inventors and advocates, but must also be demonstrably advantageous when employed in wider practice. Despite the reasonableness of this appeal, teachers profoundly influence each physician's practice. Young doctors, for example, often learn to use too many lab tests and not enough painkillers and carry these lessons into practice. The medical dictum "Never be the first to embrace a new treatment nor the last to abandon an old one" captures the speculative nature of medical innovations and the transience of conventional wisdom. This is the generational lesson alluded to by the promise to "regard my teachers as my parents."

The *Oath* now turns from ancestors to descendents.

NOTES

1. *Techné* is defined in Chapter 8.

2. Knox B. in Notes (*Sophocles* [1984] 274). Athenian law required people to support their parents.

3. Biographies of Hippocrates may be found in Jouanna 3–54, Lloyd [1979] 9–60, Carella 228–30, Temkin 52–75, Joly R. "Hippocrates of Cos" (in Gillespie 418–31).

4. Homer. Iliad II:831–5.

5. Smith 1990.

6. Jouanna 181–291.

7. Temkin 4–7, 72–5, 118–25, 183–96.

8. Temkin op cit.; Kibre P. Hippocratic writings in the Middle Ages. Bull Hist Med 1945:371–412 (esp 372).

9. Nutton B. What's in an Oath? J R Coll Physicians of Lond 1995;6:518–24.

10. This matter is discussed in chapters 2 and 7.

11. Dante Allighieri. Inferno, Canto I:72; Purgatorio, Canto xxix: 133–4; Inferno, Canto IV:34.

12. Smith (1979); Jouanna 364; Lloyd ([1991] 195, 398–416; Horstmanshoff HFJ. The ancient physician: Craftsman or scientist. J Hist Med Allied Sci 1990;45:176–97.

13. Kibre op. cit., 371–412.

14. Jouanna 364–5; Warner JH. "Making History in American Medical Culture: The Antebellum Competition for Hippocrates," in Cantor 200–5.

15. Littré.

16. Three works are commonly cited: "The Distinctive Hellenism of Greek Medicine" (367–400), "The Professional Ethics of the Greek Physician" (319–48), and "The Hippocratic Oath: Text, translation and interpretation" (4–63) All are anthologized in Temkin and Temkin, whose pagination I use.

17. Edelstein in Temkin and Temkin 345–7.

18. Edelstein in Temkin and Temkin 62–3.

19. See Pellegrino and Thomasma 124. Pellegrino 21, 111. Kass 227–8. May 100. May WF. "Code, Covenant, Contract or Philanthropy," in Veatch 2000, 117–34. Engelhardt 315. Mall D. "Death and the rhetoric of unknowing" in Horan and Mall 650. Beauchamp and McCullough 29. Rich BA. Postmodern medicine: Deconstructing the Hippocratic Oath. Univ Col Law Rev 1993;65:77–136. Zaner RM. Justice and the individual in the Hippocratic tradition. Cambridge Quarterly 1996;5:511–8. Carrick leans to authorship by persons who shared Pythagorean views but who were not necessarily Pythagoreans. He concludes that the *Oath* represents "a small and largely ignored reform movement." He follows Edelstein in taking the abortion and euthanasia passages as "all-important" and in concluding that the *Oath* is fulfilled in Christianity (Carrick 180, 94–9). In 1981, Veatch comfortably quotes the Pythagorean hypothesis ([1981] 21, 166) but by 1995 notes the controversy and takes a more skeptical position (Veatch RM, "Medical Codes and Oaths," in Reich [1995] 1420.) Jonsen is skeptical of the Pythagorean hypothesis but has not written extensively on this matter (Jonsen [2000] 8).

20. See von Staden H. "In a pure and holy way:" Personal and professional conduct in the Hippocratic Oath. J Hist Med Allied Sci 1996;51:404–37, esp. 409, notes 8–10. Kudlien F. Medical ethics and popular ethics in Greece and Rome. Clio Med 1970;5:91–121. Carrick (many sections). Jouanna (401–2). Nutton V. "Hippocratic Morality and Modern Medicine," in Flashar and Jouanna 131–63. Smith (1990, 10) takes an agnostic position. Lloyd says that the quintessential Hippocratic treatise "*On Ancient Medicine*" is a rebuttal to Pythagorean medical philosophers, suggesting a contentious dialogue with them (Lloyd [1991] 50–3). Carella accepts Edelstein's reading in its entirety (315–32).

21. Rodin.

22. Lerner extensively discusses this matter.

23. On Fractures I.

24. Nuland SB. A very wide and deep dissection. N.Y. Review of Books 2001;48:14 (Sept 20):51–3.

25. Lerner 63.

26. Lerner 108, 235.

27. Reilly BM, Hart A, Evans AT. Evidence-based medicine: a passing fancy or the future of primary care? Dis Mon 1998;44:370–99.

4

LEARNERS

[A]ND TO GIVE A SHARE BOTH OF RULES AND OF LECTURES,
AND OF ALL THE REST OF LEARNING, TO MY SONS AND TO THE
[SONS] OF HIM WHO HAS TAUGHT ME AND TO THE PUPILS WHO
HAVE SWORN BY A MEDICAL CONVENTION BUT BY NO OTHER.

In the *Oath's* opening passages, the new physician looks back to the mythic origins of medicine, enters the lineage of physicians, and assumes filial obligations to his teachers. This passage looks to its future and to the duty to transmit medical knowledge to colleagues and students of medicine. These words is notable both for the expansive definition of who should be given medical knowledge and for the extent of the information that each physician swears to share.

The physician vows to recognize the heirs of medical knowledge as including "my sons," and "the sons of him who has taught me" (a category that includes the sons of persons who were taught medicine though they did not come from a medical family), and "pupils who have sworn by a medical convention." This company of persons extends beyond the scope of one's own apprentices to encompass colleagues and apprentices other than one's own. In this opening of the profession to those who cannot claim to be descendents of Asclepius, the *Oath* explicitly breaks with the tradition of physicians as a hereditary guild.[1]

The *Oath* offers a similarly expansive definition of the medical knowledge that is to be shared as "rules," "lectures," and "all the rest of learning." The

differences between these terms may be partly inferred from differences between the kinds of information contained in the ancient medical treatises.
"Rules" seems to refer to medical precepts such as the diagnostic, therapeutic,
and prognostic inferences contained in works like *Aphorisms, Precepts,* or
Prorrhetic I. "Lectures" refers to synthetic presentations by respected teachers
as exemplified by *Prognostic, Joints,* or *Fractures.* All the rest of learning may
refer to speculations about the science of medicine as presented in works like
Ancient Medicine or *The Art.* In vowing to share this comprehensively defined
body of knowledge, the physician pledged to sustain and nurture the future of
medical learning with the insights gleaned during his own career.

These generous definitions of the heirs of medical knowledge and of the
information to be given them is quite unlike a cultic control of doctrinal secrets. Greek physicians fulfilled this obligation by offering apprenticeships,
lecturing, and writing medical treatises. This is an appropriate place to examine the nature and history of those medical writings in more detail.

THE ANCIENT MEDICAL TREATISES

The Hippocratic medical library is a diverse collection. It includes theoretical
works such as *Ancient Medicine, The Sacred Disease,* and *Waters.* There are
clinical texts such as *Aphorisms, Epidemics,* and *Wounds in the Head,* as well
as anatomical, surgical, and gynecological treatises. *Oath, Precepts, Law, Decorum,* and *Physician* are primarily works of medical ethics. Such categories
do not do justice to the diverse topics covered within each book. Some treatises discuss logistical details, such as how to equip and light a clinic or trim
one's fingernails for surgery. Case reports describe the treatment of citizens and
slaves, dying persons, and the pitfalls in undertaking the care of patients who
are incurably ill. These texts illuminate the *Oath* at least to the extent that they
describe the medical culture from which it emerged. The story of how the
ancient Greek medical treatises came to be written and then compiled into
the Hippocratic collection, transmitted, corrupted in translation, and salted with
forgeries and apocryphal works is intriguing, if murky.

The earliest treatises were written from the fifth to the early fourth century
BCE. Though the extent of literacy at that time is debated, Greece was a liter-
ate society, as evidenced by the many inscriptions on public walls and monu-
ments. Schools were in the news. In 490 BCE, a school roof collapsed, killing
all but one of the 120 students beneath it. About the same time, an enraged

athlete pushed out the supporting beam of another school roof, hurting many students. Images on graves depict young men reading scrolls. The older medical works were written during the transition from oral to recorded history. Though Greece imported its alphabet in 900 BCE, its written language was evolving while the medical works were being written. Conventions like writing from left to right were not settled until about 300 BCE, a century after the writing of many of the medical texts.[2] This partly explains why the sentence structure of the *Oath* is not known.[3] It also partly accounts for the grammatical peculiarities, including incomplete sentences in the medical works, though corrupt translations, miscopying, and reconstructions of partially obliterated material also affected this material. Many of the medical documents were written to aid a lecturer's memory. Some address an audience directly: "Having spoken about all the febrile diseases, I come now to speak about the rest."[4] Some read like bullet points for projection slides, as in passage from *Epidemics VI*: "Kindnesses to those who are ill. . . . Entrance, conversation. Position and clothing for the sick person, hair, nails, scents."[5] For all these reasons, many of these documents are somewhat raw in form.

The authors of the medical works are anonymous. It was probably so in the earliest editions to reach major libraries, because librarians carefully recorded the authors of books entering their collections.[6] It is not known why these authors did not announce their names. Anonymity does not lessen the importance of these works or their distinctive voices, however.[7] These authors were familiar with the ideas, if not the texts, of other medical writers. Some were aligned with incompletely delineated geographical or conceptual schools of thought. For example, the author of *Regimen in Acute Diseases* begins a smashing critique with this coy opening: "The authors of the work entitled *Cnidian Sentences* have correctly described the experience of patients in individual diseases . . . [but] my judgment in these matters is in many things different from their exposition."[8] The various positions taken by these anonymous authors are not simply differences between schools of thought. They reveal an embryonic medical science winnowing through ideas that would form the foundation for the science and ethics of medicine.[9] Everything was new and up for grabs.

The disputatious authors classified illnesses in a number of ways: as various imbalances or fluxes[10] of humors that were affected by age,[11] season,[12] trauma, constitution, diet, and environment.[13] Notwithstanding such differences, most authors shared the conviction that observation, rather than speculative theorizing, was the best way to nurture medical science. The distinctive voice of the author of *Ancient Medicine* (perhaps the master himself)—as grumpy and impatient as any modern medical school dean—asserts the conclusion that prevailed about the role of speculative theorizing about hot and cold humors as a form of medical science.

> I am utterly at a loss to know how those who prefer these hypothetical arguments . . . ever cure anyone. . . . I do not think they ever discovered anything that is purely "hot" or "cold," "dry" or "wet" . . . rather they impute heat to one substance, cold to another. . . . It is my opinion that all that has been written by sophists on Nature has more to do with painting than medicine.
>
> I do not believe that any clear knowledge of Nature can be obtained through any source other than a study of medicine and then only through a thorough mastery of this science. . . . Thus, if anyone were able to light upon the truth by experiment . . . he would always be able to make the best pronouncements of all.[14]

With this point of view, the sedimentation of observation upon observation built the foundation for a progressing natural science on which Western medicine would rise. The equally old treatise *Epidemic I* summarized it this way, "The physician is the servant of science."[15]

Joly says that this science was a "pre-science," a transitional phase between lore and science.[16] If so, it seems more than halfway to science in its tenet that medicine should accumulate observations that will lead to the inferences, explanations, and predictions that will be useful in healing.[17] As the author of *Ancient Medicine* said, "Full discovery will be made if the inquirer be competent, conduct his researches with knowledge of the discoveries already made and make them his starting point."[18] Many books compile associations between clinical signs and prognostic observations. Some are quite insightful:

> Blood or pus in the urine indicates ulceration of the kidneys or bladder.[19]

> Should the breasts of a woman with child suddenly become thin, she miscarries.[20]

Others, however thought-provoking, did not stand the test of time:

> Unrestrained lechery is a cure for dysentery.[21]

> For flatulence, phlebotomy.[22]

Such conclusions, with rare exception,[23] are based on observation and inference, rather than on experimental research as it is known today.[24] Without an experimental methodology to test and validate their findings or hypotheses, Greek medical science was limited to the modest accomplishment of accurate compilation.

When the medical texts use the word *experiment*, they are generally referring to when to change a therapy on a patient who is undergoing treatment. These examples are from two different works:

> Do not disturb a patient either during or just after a crisis, and try no experiments, neither with purges nor with other irritants, but leave him alone.[25]

> [If] it is clear that, of the regimen the patient is wont to use, either all, or the greater part, or some one part, is not suited to him . . . this one should learn and change . . . sometimes taking away and sometimes adding . . . and so making changes in drugging or in regimen to suit the several conditions of age, season, physique, and disease.[26]

Such experiments superficially resemble modern day "N of 1" prescriptive trials.[27] Physicians today are often uncertain whether an individual patient (who is the one subject of the N of 1 trial) will be improved by or able to tolerate a particular therapy. Accordingly, a therapy is prescribed and if suitable for that one patient it is continued; otherwise, another therapy is tried. The difference between the N = 1 empirical trial and the prescribing experiments of ancient Greece is that the efficacy of each of the modern alternatives available to a modern physician has been validated by controlled research on many patients. In Greece, the value of alternative regimens was based on an individual physicians inferences from unstructured observations.

The advent of written compilations of medical observations transformed the development of medical science. The written word facilitated reliability, accountability, and the dissemination of ideas for debate and validation. Medical education was no longer a matter of passing along an oral tradition of medical lore. Ironically, these writings could, and to some extent did, become a new kind of canonized authority that slowed medical innovation.[28] Greek physicians, for example, enthusiastically used bloodletting for many conditions. Phlebotomy persisted until the late 1800s, long outliving its rationale and even research by Pierre Louis (French physician, 1787–1872), who showed that it

did not improve survival in people with pneumonia. Even so, the reliably recorded observation is a prerequisite for research and professional accountability that the ancient Greeks greatly advanced even if they were not the first to
employ it.

CREATING THE HIPPOCRATIC COLLECTION

Collectors began acquiring the medical treatises as soon as they were written.[29]
Aristotle had a large personal library, and he and Plato were clearly familiar
with several of the medical treatises.[30] Despite such collecting, only a fraction
of the medical works survived. An inscription refers to an author of 256 medical books, of which not one remains.[31] Private collectors could only do so much.
The invention of the state-supported library was critical to the archiving, copying, translation, and survival of the ancient medical works.

The great library at Alexandria in know as Egypt is credited with the first
effort to compile and catalog the medical documents.[32] Founded in 300 BCE,
its mission was to assemble all of the world's knowledge under one roof. It's
librarians begged, borrowed, rented, and stole books from libraries throughout Europe and Asia Minor. One Hippocratic papyrus was taken from a physician whose boat docked at Alexandria.[33] Borrowed books were copied;
sometimes the original was returned to its owner.[34] Much is made of the library fire allegedly caused by Julius Caesar in 47 BCE. It destroyed 40,000
papyrus books—an immense loss, but only about five percent of the library's
collection at that time. The library remained open for another 300 years, suffering from fires, thefts, ideologically driven destruction of texts, and lack of
funds.

The earliest works were written in the Ionic dialect of the Greek language,
a dialect that differed from later Attic Greek, which was more familiar to the
treatise's compilers. For centuries, scholars of varying skill struggled to translate the Ionian Greek works into Arabic, Attic Greek, and finally into Latin.
Copies of the translations made their way throughout Greece, Rome, and
Persia. The original texts were lost.

Collectors created the idea that the written records from ancient Greece
constituted a Hippocratic Collection.[35] The documents were independently
written monographs rather a multivolume textbook of medicine. It is possible
that a few may have been written as small sets, though some scholars argue

that such groups of books (such as *Joints, Fractures,* and *Mochlicon*) were single works that became broken into separate volumes.[36] Erotian (75 CE), Galen (170 CE), and Bacchius (250 BCE) each attempted to assign authorship of particular treatises to Hippocrates or his immediate circle. In this process, Hippocrates became "the physician of record" of the ancient world.[37] Modern scholars are mostly agnostic as to which of the oldest texts Hippocrates wrote and which were written by his colleagues, but they have made some progress in classifying the treatises according to the time when editing seems to have ended.

The manuscripts were extensively recopied from the eighth through the fifteenth centuries, at which time they had become the centerpiece of medical education. For example, at the University of Caen, seventy lectures were given on the *Aphorisms* (usually accompanied with Galen's commentary), thirty-eight on the *Prognostics,* and so on.[38] Most of today's French, German, and English translations are based on manuscripts that only date to 600 to 900 CE. In other words, our versions of these texts are based on documents that underwent more than a millennium of retranslating and recopying.

The "Hippocratic library" is like an archeological dig. Five hundred years of medical civilization—from classic Greece, across the Hellenistic Age, the Roman age, to the emergence of Christianity—are compacted into a six-inch thick sediment of printed pages. Many works were pulverized and lost. Some passages were incoherently reconstructed or copied. Translators and restorers corrupted others. The repeated copying onto various papyri and moving from library to library broke some treatises apart or reassembled several treatises in new ways. Sometimes older material was inserted into newer works like an old column might be salvaged for use in a newer building. Sometimes, translators pushed new material into older works.[39]

I am unconvinced by those who argue that a coherent Hippocratic ethic can be discerned from this half-millennium of medical writings.[40] As its Greek stem *ethos* denotes, ethics is an expression of a culture. Mediterranean culture changed enormously over the 500 years during which the Hippocratic works were written. Sparta defeated Athens. Athenians' confidence was shaken during the ensuing governmental instability. Rome conquered Greece. A two-hundred-year gap between groups of treatises shrouds the historical continuity of these works (see Appendix A). As the late treatises, such as the ethics work *Decorum,* were being written, Christian morality was supplanting the Greek ethics. An assertion of constancy of medical ethics from when the *Oath* was written in 400 BCE through Roman and even early Christian-era texts must be proven rather than presumed. This book focuses on Greek medical writings that are contemporaneous with the writing of the *Oath*: those that are believed to have been written between 450 and 350 BCE.[41] At that time, Hippocrates was either living or in living memory.

✻   ✻   ✻

CASE 4.1 The chief resident asked me to speak about the diagnosis of dementia at "Doughnut Rounds." These lectures are named for morning conferences at which doughnuts are served. A drug company usually hosts the affair and supplies food. On the table next to the food, the host places trinkets promoting the sponsor's products. These might be notepads, simple medical equipment, toy animals to hang on stethoscopes, or plastic pocket treatment guidelines that invariably suggest prescribing the drug company's products. The salesperson passes out promotional literature and research papers (usually reprints of studies that were funded by the hosting company) that showcase the company's products. The residents filed into the room and took ten minutes to pick up the trinkets, literature and food. The chief resident thanked the sponsor. Then the drug salesperson spoke for a couple minutes promoting his blood pressure medicine. He did not mention that impartial experts recommend other, less expensive drugs made by competing companies. Then I was introduced and gave my lecture.

The sales attention lavished on Doughnut Rounds is a small part of the $13,000 per physician that drug companies spend every year to promote the prescription of their products.[42] The larger effort includes buying physicians dinners, trips to resorts, and supplying free samples of drugs (many of which physicians and their staff take for personal use[43]). Once a liposuction manufacturer offered me a trip to Mexico to learn how to use its equipment and guaranteed I would be able to practice on two patients while I was there!

Interns, residents, and medical students attend from two to seventy Doughnut Rounds each year. They also receive up to hundreds of dollars worth of gifts, dinners and concerts. Young physicians are those most heavily exposed and the least prepared to recognize the bias in drug salespersons' presentations. They are also less insightful into the effect that such promotional presentations have on their practice.[44] They come to rely on sales representatives for information that they should obtain from a balanced reading of the medical literature.[45]

Information presented by salespeople at Doughnut Rounds is biased.[46] They overstate the clinical advantages and roles of newer, more expensive drugs, minimize the side effects of their medications, and fail to mention comparably effective, often less expensive therapies. Their handouts are typically sales brochures or summarize company-sponsored research.[47] About half the sales brochures fail to meet government standards for fairness or validate their claims; ten percent of the claims in sales brochures are inaccurate. Not surprisingly, such misstatements favor the promoted product.[48] This kind of "education" does not promote good habits for lifelong learning. Neither does it serve patients' best interests.

The sales effort that is aimed at physicians profoundly shapes their clinical decisions.[49] Gifts and social contacts make young doctors eight times as likely to prescribe a second-best drug when alternative therapies are better. Senior physicians who socialize with and accept money from drug salespeople are ten to twenty times as likely to ask that a new drug be added to a hospital pharmacy. When patients learn how drug salespeople use gifts and biased material to shape medical practice, their respect for physicians and medical schools diminishes considerably. Patients are likelier than physicians to believe that such sales contacts raise the cost of health while lowering the quality of care.[50] Calls for reform or abolition of education by drug representatives have largely gone unheeded.

How might the vow "to give a share both of rules and of lectures, and of all the rest of learning" to one's students and colleagues apply to Doughnut Rounds? It seems reasonable to conclude that this passage speaks to the deans and professors of medical schools who have shouldered the role of teaching the next generation of physicians. Students and residents are successors to the medical apprentices of ancient Greece. Similarly, the physician employees of drug companies who craft the information for salespeople to present are also engaged in imparting knowledge to physicians.

Second, the words "I swear by Apollo . . . to give a share both of rules and of lectures, and of all the rest of learning" sound like a modern oath to "speak the truth, the whole truth and nothing but the truth, so help me, God." In the sense of the *Oath's* definition of medical information, those who would teach physicians must pledge to impart accurate, fair, and complete medical information. The research cited above suggests that Doughnut Rounds do not meet this standard.

Finally, the passage on imparting medical knowledge is integrally related to the *Oath's* larger message that physicians are fundamentally committed to "benefit the ill" and avoid harmful injustice. By contrast, Doughnut Rounds are primarily designed to increase the sales and market share of particular treatments even when other therapies are less expensive or more appropriate.[51] The *Oath* binds the content and aims of medical education to the interests of patients in a manner that conflicts with content and aims presented by the sponsors of Doughnut Rounds.

NOTES

1. Jouanna 47–48.
2. Casson 17–30. Lloyd (1991) 124. Humez and Humez.
3. von Staden H. "In a pure and holy way": Personal and professional conduct in the Hippocratic Oath. J Hist Med Allied Sci 1996;51:406–8.
4. For example, see *Diseases III:1* and *Nature of Man 1.*
5. *Epidemics* 6;4:7.
6. Casson 35. The treatises were also harshly critical of other unnamed physicians, temple healers, and philosophers; however, it was not customary to name persons whom one criticized (Jouanna 280.).
7. Smith (1979) 30.
8. *Regimen in Acute Diseases I* (Hippocrates 1950).
9. Lloyd GER. The transformations of ancient medicine. Bull Hist Med 1992; 66:114–32.
10. *Places in Man (many references).*
11. *Aphorisms III:24–31.*
12. *Aphorisms III:20–3.*
13. *Humours 12.* See Carella 286–313 and Jouanna 146–54.
14. *Tradition in Medicine 1, 15, 20, 24.* Translation from Hippocrates 1950. Loeb title of same treatise is *On Ancient Medicine.*
15. *Epidemics I:ii(11) Translation from Hippocrates 1950.*
16. Joly R. "Hippocrates of Cos," in Gillespie. 418–31.
17. Riddle JM. "Folk Tradition and Folk Medicine: Recognition of Drugs in Classical Antiquity" (in Scarborough, 22–61) offers a comprehensive index to these therapies.

18. *On Ancient Medicine II.*

19. *Aphorisms IV;lxxv.*

20. *Aphorisms V;xxxvii.*

21. *Epidemics 7:122.*

22. *Epidemics 2.5.5.*

23. This is one of the few real experiments described in the Greek medical works. "One may put twenty eggs or more to hatch under two hens and each day, beginning on the second day . . . take away an egg and break it open: one will discover by examination that everything agrees with what I have said (about fetal development, membranes, and the fetal cord.) (*Nature of Child* 29 Translation from Hippocrates, 1950)

24. Lloyd (1991) 70–99, 110–20.

25. *Aphorisms I:xx.*

26. *Nature of Man: IX.* See also *The Art: xi.*

27. Guyatt GH, Keller JL, Jaeschke R et al. The N-of-1 randomized controlled trial: Clinical usefulness. Ann Intern Med 1990;112:293–9.

28. Lloyd (1983) 115–35, 202.

29. Casson 26–30. Plato tells us that copies of Anaxagoras's treatise on cosmology cost one drachma in the market—affordable to the élite; a day's wage for working people. (Plato. *Apology* 26:d).

30. Joly R. "Hippocrates and the School of Cos," in Gillespie 29–48, Mansfeld J. "The Historical Hippocrates and the Origins of Scientific Medicine, " in Ruse 49–75. See also Casson 31.

31. Drabkin IE. Medical education in ancient Greece and Rome. Bull Hist Med 1944;15:333–51 at 350.

32. Casson 31–47.

33. Basbanes 63.

34. Smith (1979) 200–1.

35. Lloyd (1991) 205–22.

36. Jouanna 373–416.

37. Smith WD. Notes on ancient medical historiography. Bull Hist Med 1989; 63:73–109. Carrick 76–80. Carella 231–3.

38. Kibre P. Hippocratic writings in the Middle Ages. Bull Hist Med 1945:371–412.

39. Most of the translators comment on this issue and highlight various unintelligible or corrupted passages. For example, see Smith ([1990] 43); Jones ([1923] iii–iv); and Hanson AE. "Continuity and Change: Three Case Studies in Hippocratic Gynecological Therapy and Theory," in Pomeroy (1991) 73–110.

40. For example, Owsei Temkin writes, "A quotation from the works of Hippocrates, literal or paraphrased, a theory or practice ascribed to him by one or another author will be taken as representing Hippocratic medicine. . . . Most of the Hippocratic works were probably written between the late fifth and the middle of the fourth century BC. The fact that a few books written around the first century AD were incorporated into the Hippocratic Collection is proof enough that there was no hiatus between the old and the new." ([1991], ix–xi.) Carrick also accepts the constancy of the Hippocratic tradition from the sixth through the first centuries BCE (Carrick 5).

41. I accept Langhoff (36) on this point. The differences between the texts of this narrower time frame are matters of different views held by cosmopolitan physicians who were influenced by each other within a single cultural milieu. By focusing on the early works, I accept the loss of ideas in treatises written several hundred years after Hippocrates. Minimizing the introduction of Hellenistic and Roman thinking in these later works offsets this loss.

42. Henry J. Kaiser Family Foundation. Trends and Indicators in the Changing Health Care Marketplace, 2002. May 2002, Menlo Park, CA. http://www.kff.org/content/2002/3254/GluckFinalReportweb3254.pdf

43. Westfall JM, McCabe J, Nicholas RA. Personal use of drug samples by physicians and office staff. JAMA 1997;278:141–3.

44. Hodges B. Interactions with the pharmaceutical industry: Experiences and attitudes of psychiatry residents, interns and clerks. CMAJ 1995;153:553–9. McKinney WP, Scheidermayer DL, Lurie N, et al. Attitudes of internal medicine faculty and residents toward professional interaction with pharmaceutical sales representatives. JAMA 1990;264:1693–7. Steinman MA, Shlipak MG, McPhee SJ. Of principles and pens: Attitudes and practices of medicine housestaff toward pharmaceutical industry promotions. Am J Med 2001;110:551–7.

45. Spingarn RW, Berlin JA, Strom BL. When pharmaceutical manufacturers' employees present grand rounds, what do residents remember? Acad Med 1996; 71:86–8. Lurie N, Rich EC, Simpson DE, et al. Pharmaceutical representatives in academic medical centers: Interaction with faculty and housestaff. J Gen Intern Med 1990;5:240–3.

46. Ziegler MG, Lew P, Singer BC. The accuracy of drug information from pharmaceutical sales representatives. JAMA 273:1296–8.

47. See Chapter 9 on "In a pure and holy way . . . " for a discussion of corporate-sponsored research.

48. Stryer D, Bero LA. Characteristics of materials distributed by drug companies: An evaluation of appropriateness. J Gen Intern Med 1996;11:575–83.

49. Spingarn RW, Berlin JA, Strom BL. When pharmaceutical manufacturers' employees present grand rounds, what do residents remember? Acad Med. 1996;71:86–8.

Dieperink ME, Drogemuller L. Industry-sponsored grand rounds and prescribing behavior. JAMA 2000;285:1443–4. Tenery RM. Interactions between physicians and the health care technology industry. JAMA 2000;283:391–3. Wazana A. Physicians and the pharmaceutical industry: Is a gift ever just a gift? JAMA 2000;283:373–80. Orlowski JP, Wateska L. The effects of pharmaceutical firm enticements on physician prescribing patterns: There is no such thing as a free lunch. Chest 1992;102:270–3.

50. Gibbons RV, Landry FJ, Blouch DL, et al. A comparison of physicians' and patients' attitudes toward pharmaceutical industry gifts. J Gen Intern Med 1998; 13:151–4. Mainous AG III, Hueston WJ, Rich EJ. Patients' perceptions of physician acceptance of gifts from the pharmaceutical industry. Arch Fam Med 1995; 4:335–9. Blake RL Jr, Early EK. Patients' attitudes about gifts to physicians from pharmaceutical companies. J Am Board Fam Pract 1995;8:457–64.

51. Wall LL, Brown D. Pharmaceutical sales representatives and the doctor/patient relationship. Obstet Gynecol 2002;100:594–9.

II

TO WHAT ARE
PHYSICIANS COMMITTED?

I WILL USE REGIMENS FOR THE BENEFIT OF THE ILL IN
ACCORDANCE WITH MY ABILITY AND MY JUDGMENT, BUT FROM
WHAT IS TO THEIR HARM OR INJUSTICE I WILL KEEP THEM.

I WILL NOT GIVE A DRUG THAT IS DEADLY TO ANYONE IF
ASKED FOR IT, NOR WILL I SUGGEST THE WAY TO SUCH A
COUNSEL.

AND LIKEWISE I WILL NOT GIVE A WOMAN A DESTRUCTIVE
PESSARY.

IN A PURE AND HOLY WAY I WILL GUARD MY LIFE AND MY
TECHNÉ.

I WILL NOT CUT, AND CERTAINLY NOT THOSE SUFFERING
FROM STONE, BUT I WILL CEDE THIS TO MEN WHO ARE
PRACTITIONERS OF THIS ACTIVITY.

INTO AS MANY HOUSES AS I MAY ENTER, I WILL GO FOR THE
BENEFIT OF THE ILL, WHILE BEING FAR FROM ALL VOLUNTARY
AND DESTRUCTIVE INJUSTICE, ESPECIALLY FROM SEXUAL ACTS
BOTH UPON WOMEN'S BODIES AND UPON MEN'S, BOTH OF THE
FREE AND OF THE SLAVES.

ABOUT WHATEVER I MAY SEE OR HEAR IN TREATMENT, OR
EVEN WITHOUT TREATMENT, IN THE LIFE OF HUMAN BEINGS—
THINGS THAT SHOULD NOT EVER BE BLURTED OUT OUTSIDE—
I WILL REMAIN SILENT, HOLDING SUCH THINGS TO BE
UNUTTERABLE [SACRED, NOT TO BE DIVULGED].

The health-care professions are so deeply integrated into modern Western societies that it is easy to overlook the terms of the special ethical "contract" for their conduct. With the consent of the patient, a physician may inquire about virtually any aspect of a person's life and may touch any part of the body. Physicians may cut on living persons and dissect human corpses. They may disclose an impending death, write prescriptions for drugs that can kill, and then certify the cause of death of the same persons who have taken those drugs. They are permitted to have a personal financial stake in treatment decisions and in the outcome of the research that they conduct. The legal and ethical norms for these activities and many others are governed by an implicit or explicit pact between physicians and society.

Each provision of this pact has been debated. Each has been controversial. Some provisions, such as the duty to tell a patient that he or she has contracted a terminal disease, are new to our culture. Others, such as donating one's body for dissection, have been negotiated within the past hundred years or so. Others are much older. Each provision is shaped by diverse and evolving cultural norms. In the United States, unlike some countries, a physician may counsel and treat a person without obtaining the approval of a clan leader. In many parts of the world, physicians must seek the consent of a women's husband before giving her treatment or information.

The passages of the *Oath* discussed in Part II are a physician's proclamation of commitments to society and to patients. This is neither a comprehensive list of all the norms that applied to Greek physicians nor a code of law. Before considering each passage individually, it is worthwhile to examine how these passages are organized to form a larger argument about the physician in Greek society and in the clinical encounter.

Ancient Greece distinguished between public and private spheres of life. Some scholars argue that this distinction, which emerged about 520 BCE, was a crowning Greek invention in that it was fundamental to the idea of democracy.[1] *Democracy*, "rule by the people," is premised on the idea that the prerogatives of government and of private life may be separated. To make this possible, a new political role, *citizenship*, was created.[2] Thus, in defining the *polis* as a democratic state, the Greeks simultaneously defined the *political* ("that which affects everybody") and *politai* ("citizens"). As citizens came to expect to be free of despotic intrusions, they could create a private sphere that their political engagement made possible.[3] Among the paradigmatic crimes of the despotic Thirty Tyrants (404–403 BCE) was breaking into citizen's houses—a violation of the boundaries between the public and private spheres.[4] The naming of this crime occurred at about the time when the *Oath* was written. These public and private spheres were partly spatially defined. The "house," *oikia*, was the fundamental unit of Greek society, which to some extent demarked the private space. A house was both a social and a physical space. It consisted of the dwelling, a family, its lineage, possessions, and social position. Crimes and their punishments varied according to where acts were performed. For example, stealing a coat in the market was an offence against society and differed from stealing a coat from a home (where personal revenge or a civil lawsuit were more likely to be the appropriate responses). In short, the concept of *public* and *private* was important to the culture, its sense of governance, its sense of home life, and in distinguishing various kinds of transgressions.

The *Oath* reflects this sense of the public and the private spheres.[5] It seems to have two "stanzas": one speaking of the ethics of public medical life, the second describing the ethics of the physician in the patient's private world in which the clinical encounter occurred.[6] (See Table II. 1.) Three pieces of evidence support this stanzaic organization.

First, the organization of each stanza mirrors the other. Each invokes the principles of beneficence and the promise to reject injustice and then lists two transgressions.

Second, the public medical ethic precedes passages describing the medical ethics in the patient's private world. This continues the *Oath's* progression from general to specific. The *Oath's* initial passages, discussed in Part I, speak of the profession's origins and its regard for teachers and students. The passages pertaining to the physician in society define principles, "benefit" and "justice," which are illustrated with two exemplary taboos. The first taboo refers to deadly drugs and the second to abortive pessaries. This order seems counter-intuitive from a modern perspective on medical ethics that tends to follow a life-course in which the abortion precedes euthanasia just as the beginning of life precedes actions at end of life. As we shall see, however, this order makes sense in the context of the *Oath's* progression from the social to the personal. The first taboo speaks to the general societal fear of the physician-poisoner; the second is a vow to the head of the household just before the physician enters the patient's house to not interfere with his authority over reproduction in the house. Following these taboos and a puzzling passage on cutting for stone, the physician purifies himself, enters the patient's house, and the *Oath* becomes very personal. Within the house, the principles of benefit and justice are proposed in a different way, and two more taboos are given as examples of how these principles may violated. These taboos pertain to sexual relations with members of the house and dishonorably speaking of the private matters of the inhabitants.

The public and private taboos strikingly differ in the degree to which they are personalized. Both assert that "benefiting" the ill and "avoiding injustice" are fundamental principles for medical care, but this reiteration is not a simple refrain. The public stanza uses "benefiting the ill" and "injustice" impersonally and refers to protecting the ill from injustice (implicitly inflicted by others). By contrast, in the clinical ethics stanza, the physician vows to personally refrain from treating a patient in an unjust manner. Another aspect of the personalization is the opening phrase of this stanza, "Into as many houses as I may enter." "I enter" (and its reiterating "I will go") are the only verbs in the *Oath* that are not used in relation to moral pledges or moral assessments. In this theatrical movement,[7] the moral attention of the physician turns from the public to private world. In that private world, persons have gender and social

TABLE II.1 Public and Private Ethics Stanzas

	Ethics of the Public Sphere	*Ethics of the Private Sphere*
Principles (benefit, injustice)	I will use regimens for the *benefit* of the ill in accordance with my ability and my judgment, but from what is to their harm or *injustice* I will keep them.	Into as many houses as I may enter, I will go for the *benefit* of the ill, while being far from all voluntary and destructive *injustice*,
First example	I will not give a drug that is deadly to anyone if asked for it, nor will I suggest the way to such a counsel.	Especially from sexual acts both upon women's bodies and upon men's, both of the free and of the slaves.
Second example	Likewise, I will not give a woman a destructive pessary.	About whatever I may see or hear in treatment, or even without treatment, in the life of human beings—things that should not ever be blurted out outside—I will remain silent, holding such things to be unutterable [sacred, not to be divulged].

rank, and the intimate acts of sexual relations in a patient's house and revealing personal secrets are named.

Medical ethics today still distinguishes between clinical ethics and the ethics of the physician in society. Clinical ethics focuses on the personal duties of the physician–patient relationship, including such issues as respecting informed consent, not having sex with patients, terminating the clinical relationship, and the rules for discussing care with family or for informing the patient about how medical information will be shared with others. The ethics of medicine in society include issues like the physician's role in capital punishment, health-care reform, and so on. One must be cautious in analogizing between the topics addressed by the public and private medical ethics of Greece and those of today, given the differences between these cultures.

NOTES

1. Meier 53–81.

2. A full discussion of the public and private spheres goes far beyond the scope of this book. Though many authors allude to it, the most complete and illuminating discussion that I found was in Meier.

3. Cohen (1991) 70–97. Patterson C 70–106, 180–225.

4. Cohen (1995) 53.

5. Vivian Nutton agrees with this division and its demarcation by the entry into the house (personal correspondence with SM, 12/20/02).

6. Kass divides the *Oath* into topical paragraphs: he calls the sections that I include in the Public Ethic plus the surgical passage "Treatment paragraphs" and the sections that I call the Private Ethics Stanza "Decorum paragraphs." He arrives at this distinction by dividing the *Oath* into paragraphs that he groups into topics, though he writes, "I hasten to add that this distinction between treatment . . . and decorum is foreign to the text" (Kass 229). I believe that Kass' organization breaks down when one considers the problems of the apparent redundancy of benefit and justice and the structural problem posed by the oddly placed surgical passage. Von Staden says that *Oath* does not have decipherable punctuation. ("In a pure and holy way": Personal and professional conduct in the Hippocratic Oath. J Hist Med Allied Sci 1996;51:406–8). My view is that the *Oath* is more than just a list of promises and that we must examine it in light of the heuristic principles of its time.

7. There is an intriguing similarity between this use of movement, and stage directions to a chorus in a Greek drama to move and face a different direction. In Greek drama, such directions often marked a shift between choral stanzas (strophe and

antistrophe) that conveyed two positions on a moral issue. The relationship of the *Oath* to drama and poetry is not known. Many of the Greek medical treatises show evidence of a metric structure reflecting their proximity to the development of Greek poetic writing (Cohen [1991] 12–3). Von Staden notes that one of the canonical versions of the *Oath* has a meter but he does not relate this to the argument of the *Oath* (von Staden H. "In a pure and holy way": Personal and professional conduct in the Hippocratic Oath. J Hist Med Allied Sci 1996;51:406–8, at note 4 referring to the *Oath* in dactylic hexameters. Heiberg JL. Hippocratics Opera, Corpus Medicorums Graecorum, I Berlin/Leipzig: Teubner, 1927, pp. 4–5).

5

THE HEALTH OF THE PUBLIC

I WILL USE TREATMENTS FOR THE BENEFIT OF THE ILL IN
ACCORDANCE WITH MY ABILITY AND MY JUDGMENT BUT FROM
WHAT IS TO THEIR HARM OR INJUSTICE I WILL KEEP THEM.

Most bioethicists maintain that the *Oath* proposes a clinical ethic that is centered on the direct treatment of a patient and does not address the physician's moral engagement with the broader society. Edelstein, for example, maintained that medical ethics in ancient Greece was simply bedside etiquette and that philosophers articulated the first clinical ethic with the *Oath*.[1] Veatch describes Hippocratic ethics as "ultra-individualism" in its support for the professional autonomy of each physician. He says that the way that modern medical ethics hold physicians accountable to societal norms, such as the doctrine of informed consent, "essentially overturned the core ethical positions of the Hippocratic tradition."[2] Pellegrino says the Hippocratic ethic "notably [contains] no sense of the larger responsibilities as a profession for the behavior of each member. Nowhere stated are the potentialities and responsibilities of a group of high minded individuals to effect reforms and achieve purposes transcending the interests of individual members."[3]

Such personal isolation from a sense of civic duty would have been an unusual claim for citizens of Greek city-states.[4] The ancient Greek leader Pericles described a *citizen* this way:

There is visible in the same person an attention to their own private concerns
and those of the public and in others engaged in the labors of life. There is a
competent skill in the affairs of government. For we are the only people who
think him that does not meddle in state affairs—is not indolent, but is good for
nothing.[5]

As citizens in this sense, physicians were engaged in a new craft, one that
potentially conflicted with Greek laws, traditions, heads of families and political authorities. In addition to treating patients, Greek physicians performed a
variety of civic roles. Medical treatises discussed their work with armies. Such
work goes back at least as far Homer, who said of military surgeons, "A man
who can cut out shafts and dress our wounds—a good healer is worth a troop
of other men."[6] During Hippocrates' time, physicians may have accepted dip-
lomatic missions with the understanding that the physician–citizenship role
promoted the health of the citizens of a city-state, just as clinical work promoted
the health of individuals.[7] Physicians treated people during epidemics and may
have organized public-health responses to civic health disasters.[8] Councils
appointed some physicians "city physicians."[9] Physicians, like other citizens,
would have been expected to participate in public debates about the governance
of Greek society.

Civic participation is one thing; a professional ethic that concerns potential
areas of moral engagement between professionals and society is quite another.
The possibility that Greek medical ethics was simply about clinical ethics and
bedside etiquette must be kept in mind as the *Oath* is examined for evidence
that it spoke of the civic responsibilities of physician or of norms to address
professional conflicts with the social order. Today we tend to describe societal
ethics using words like *human rights*, *fairness*, and *justice*.

GREEK JUSTICE: *DIKÉ*

Today, *justice* is usually thought of as a form of fairness that is guaranteed by
rights that are defined in some form of explicitly stated or implicitly accepted
social contract. There is procedural fairness; e.g., every person charged with a
crime is entitled to a competent legal defense. There is the justice of treating
equal cases are equally, e.g., all persons who can pay have a right to be served
at a public restaurant. There is compensatory justice that adjusts for those who

are most disadvantaged, i.e., a person with dyslexia must be allowed extra time to take a test. Unfairness is seen as harmful to individuals and to the social cohesion of the community.[10] This sense of justice as implying equal opportunity, equal rights, and redress of social disadvantages is a relatively recent formulation.

Diké is the word in the *Oath* that is currently translated as *justice*. This is a difficult translation, because ancient Greece had a different concept of justice than our sense of justice as "fairness." For this reason, older translations rendered this word as not *doing wrong* or *causing injury*.[11] In ancient Greece, acting justly meant acting in a way that comported with the ethical foundation underlying the social and natural world. In this sense, justice meant respect for moral traditions and norms for civic relationships.[12] This sense of justice accepted what we would call an unfair inequality of rights between freemen and slaves or men and women because it reflected support for existing social institutions defining one's station in life. As the Chorus in *Oedipus the King* says:

> Great laws tower above us, reared on high, borne for the brilliant vault of heaven—Olympian Sky their only father, nothing mortal, no man gave them birth, their memory deathless, never lost in sleep: within them lives a mighty god, the god does not grow old.[13]

Olympian gods did not invent this moral order, but they taught it to humans. Tradition, family, and law transmitted this moral order to succeeding generations. Sophocles gave these words to the character of Antigone, who faced execution for violating a regal proclamation and performing traditional burial honors for her slain, traitorous brother. She distinguishes between human laws and the justice of moral traditions:

> Of course [I broke the law.] It wasn't Zeus, not in the least, who made this proclamation—not to me. Nor did that Justice, dwelling with the gods beneath the earth, ordain such laws for men. Nor did I think your [King Creon's] edict had such force that you, a mere mortal, could override the gods, the great unwritten, unshakable traditions. They are alive, not just today or yesterday: they live forever, from the first of time and no one knows when they first saw the light.[14]

This organic view of "living" laws was used by Greek philosophers who saw in the homeostatic harmony of medicine's bodily humors a metaphor for how justice arose as a healthy balance between the virtues and desire.[15] Having taught the various forms of *diké* to humans, the Olympian gods retreated and left humans responsible for passing them down. This responsibility raised a new moral problem.

Why should an individual or a society strive for justice when to act justly was often an obstacle to an immediate boon? Aristotle answered that a society should pursue justice because justice engenders a world in which people can most fully flourish and find true happiness.[16] But a second question probes deeper into human responsibility in an unjust world. Even if one's own actions can be said to be just, is there a duty to act on behalf of those who have suffered injustice at the hands of others? Euripides posed this question with these words by Creusa, who was favored in life and then enslaved by war: "Where shall we appeal for justice when the injustice of power is our destruction?"[17] The *Oath's* words, "from what is to their harm or injustice I will keep them" seem to speak to Creusa's question. If they do, the *Oath* directs the physician's moral attention beyond the clinical relationship to an encounter with larger powers.

A medical ethic that is narrowly focused on clinical work would not engage the physician in matters of social injustice. Context sheds further light on the *Oath's* meaning. The vow to "keep the ill from injustice" is paired with a vow to act "for the benefit of the ill." One could argue that keeping the ill from injustice and benefiting the ill are simply two ways of saying the same thing— that a physician is duty-bound to heal the sick. This seems unlikely for three reasons. First, "injustice" is a moral transgression and thus quite unlike the affliction of a natural physical illness. This passage speaks of a physician's duty to see that the ill are not harmed by that moral transgression. Second, it seems quite unlikely that the parsimoniously written *Oath* would use "benefit the ill" and "injustice" to make a single point—that the physician should cure disease. Finally, the *Oath* has two "justice and benefit" passages, and the differences between them illuminate their separate meanings. These differences can be seen more clearly by juxtaposing them:

1. I will use treatments for the benefit of the ill in accordance with my ability and my judgment but from what is to their harm or injustice I will keep them.
2. Into as many houses as I may enter, I will go for the benefit of the ill, while being far from all voluntary and destructive injustice.

Up to the first use of "justice and benefit," the *Oath* has been speaking of the larger world of gods, teachers, and teaching. The ensuing pledge to keep the ill from injustice seems to be a promise to protect patients from a health-harming injustice by others. By contrast, the second pledge to refrain from voluntary and destructive injustice follows a passage describing a physician entering a patient's house. In this private place, it describes a promise to personally abstain from acting unjustly during the clinical encounter. Unfortunately, there is scant evidence from ancient Greece as to the kinds of physicians' duties that are commended by swearing to keep a person from injustice.

Part of the reason for this scanty record is that Athenian dramas, an aborted abolitionist movement, and some political statements suggest that in Athens the cultural debate about what we would recognize as social justice was inchoate. Pericles, for example, said, "We all enjoy the same general equality our laws are fitted to preserve. . . . The public administration is not confined to a particular family but is attainable only by merit."[18] Clearly the laws were not fitted to preserve the general equality of slaves, women, or aliens, though Greeks society did recognize the mistreatment of slaves. In a liberal spirit, the *Oath* opened medical education to any man who would properly swear and contract to undertake a medical career regardless of whether he was a son of a healer. The *Oath* also establishes a single standard for sexual relations with either freemen or slaves during clinical visits. The *Oath's* words on deadly drugs and abortive pessaries immediately follow the first passage on benefit and justice. Perhaps they can shed additional light on how the *Oath* articulated physicians' duties to *diké* and the social order.

*   *   *

CASE 5.1 In 1999, I gave a talk at a senior citizens center on geriatric medicine in a small town on the Minnesota–Canadian border. At the end of the talk, an older woman approached me privately. "Dr. Miles, I would like to ask you a question. My husband and I are on the same blood thinner. We share those pills— each of us gets half a dose because we cannot afford the two prescriptions. But, what I really want to ask you is this: I have both congestive heart failure and breast cancer, for which I am on two costly medicines. I cannot afford them both and am planning to stop taking one of them. So, I'd like your opinion on which one to stop. Is it less painful to die of breast cancer or congestive heart failure?"

The United States' system for providing basic health care covers too few people and costs too much. More than forty million Americans do not have public or private health insurance for more than one year at a time.[19] A fifth of these are children. Clinics turn away people with high blood pressure and other chronic conditions even as hospitals are required to treat the strokes, heart attacks, and other medical emergencies caused by those same untreated chronic diseases. The United States spends far more per person on health care than other nations, and costs are rising much faster than the general rate of inflation. More than 300,000 families each year identify health-care debts as the primary cause of personal bankruptcy. Medical debts deter people from seeking needed health care. The high cost of care is seen as precluding universal insurance, as all health-care sectors add to its burdens with more than a hundred billion dollars of excess administrative costs and hundreds of millions of dollars for legislative lobbying, campaign donations, and advertising. As the only industrialized nation that does not assure every citizen affordable access to basic health care, it is not surprising that the United States ranks poorly on measures of longevity, rates of disability, and infant death rates.[20]

U.S. physicians have generally organized *against* efforts to address the lack of affordable health care. They have opposed reforms proposed by Franklin Delano Roosevelt, Harry Truman, and Dwight Eisenhower. In 1965, physicians fought the passage of Medicare. With deep divisions in their ranks, physicians failed to unite in support of health-care reform during the first term of the Clinton administration.[21] To be fair, the United States' unique failure to provide universal health insurance is the result of legislative votes rather than being a situation imposed by the medical profession. Even so, the question remains: Do physicians have responsibilities that extend beyond those of competently and ethically treating patients to a duty to improve social systems, like universal health insurance, that improve the public health?

In general, engaging a civic problem like unjust access to health care is seen as a praiseworthy, but not obligatory, medical activity. Most people and physicians would agree that it is commendable for physicians to address public health threats like AIDS, provide free care, work on health-care reform, or volunteer at charity clinics in their own country or abroad. Yet a physician incurs no opprobrium for choosing to lead a competent professional life in a local clinic while leaving matters of social injustice that harms the public health to others. The American Medical Association says that each physician has an obligation to provide some free care to "the indigent," and that physicians as a group (but not each physician) should work with policymakers to help society meet its obligation to make adequate health care available to all.[22] Institutionally, the AMA has worked against universal health care and sharply criticized professional medical organizations that have broken ranks with their positions on this matter. What did this debate look like in ancient Greece?

Greek dramas depict a moral concern about the injustice of poverty as a barrier to health care.[23] In Euripides' *Electra*, a peasant laments, "What a power there is in money! You can entertain a guest; or if you're ill, buy medicine and cure yourself." Later, Electra asks her mother to perform rituals to mark the official birth of a ten-day-old boy. Her mother says, "It is usually done by the woman who delivered you." Electra replies, "I was alone, I delivered myself. . . . We are poor."[24] The satirical Aristophanes writes: "What doctor is there now left in town? There is no money to be offered so there's no medicine practiced."[25] Even so, the historical evidence about Asclepian temple practices, the function of city physicians, and charity care is simply inadequate to support any definite conclusion about the provision of medical care to indigent people in ancient Greece. There is a glimmer of a hint. Athens gave disabled veterans, incapacitated workers, and orphans who were under eighteen years old a regular allowance of funds for food and shelter.[26] Such assistance was a self-evidently effective form of life-sustaining care.

The evidence of how ancient Greek physicians viewed their personal obligation to poor patients is similarly unclear. People from all walks of life sought out and paid Greek physicians for health care. Cobblers, vine tenders, shepherds, athletes and their trainers, soldiers, potters, prostitutes, stonecutters, grooms, boxers, shopkeepers, cooks, mineworkers, masseuses, carpenters, slaves, ship captains, schoolteachers, butchers, laborers, servants, traveling salespeople—all appear as patients in the ancient medical treatises. Some were wealthier than others. Plato and the author of *Regimen III* accept that more extensive care would be given to people who wanted and could afford it.[27] Medical writings about free care and sliding-scale fees do not appear until centuries later, in Roman-era medical treatises, although earlier writings discussing such matters may have been lost.[28] In sum, the *Oath's* words about keeping the ill from injustice, the words of Greek playwrights, and the ancient Greek medical treatises all suggest that there was a moral dimension to the encounter between physicians and health-harming injustices, though there is no evidence of intellectual closure on the nature of the corresponding medical ethic to address these issues. The issues were joined but the debate was not finished. It was bequeathed to us.

Nearly every clinician today knows of patients who are humiliated, injured, or receive delayed treatment because of the way health care is financed in the United States.[29] Many clinicians have encountered people like the woman who asked me the heart-stopping question about which of her unaffordable, life-saving medications to discontinue. Most physicians will suggest a social worker to help refer such a person to a public or private program that will pay for the treatment. In this case, I knew of a new program to cover this kind of expense. Physicians also dispense free samples of medicine that drug salespeople have given them. Some people with chronic diseases like asthma repeatedly consent to be research subjects in order to obtain medications and medical attention. I once asked a cardiologist whether a well-tested, older, and less expensive combination of generic drugs might be substituted for a patient of his who could not afford the new therapy that he had prescribed. He replied, "It is my job to recommend the best and most current therapy. It would be wrong to prescribe any less." Collectively, these approaches are an unreliable, cumbersome patchwork of solutions for the many people who cannot afford medical treatment. Relatively few physicians work on the politicized area of health-care reform.

Healers could see "I will use treatments for the benefit of the ill in accordance with my ability and my judgment but from what is to their harm or injustice I will keep them" as a commitment to a medical ethic that looks outward to improve the public health by engaging public policy that unjustly harms health. Such a vow speaks with regard for those who are under the threat of harm from a moral transgression—injustice. This medical ethic would look beyond the clinical attention to one's own patients to the way that people's health is affected by the larger world. The implications of this moral vision for professional action should evolve with the scientific understanding of public health threats, just as clinical treatment evolved since ancient Greece with our understanding of how to treat individual patients.

This understanding of the *Oath* has discernible roots in the medical ethics debates of ancient Greece, and it fits into the evolving medial ethics of our time. Medical associations have promulgated strong positions condemning any individual physician or medical association that collaborates with or conceals torture.[30] Physicians have addressed the threat to public health posed by weapons of mass destruction and international economic sanctions.[31] The broader relationship between medical ethics and human rights is also being explored.[32] There are international standards that apply to all physicians for protecting human subjects of biomedical research.[33] The lack of clear engagement by United States physicians in working with public and civic institutions to address the consequences of harms caused by unjust health-care financing is part of the crisis of trust confronting the medical profession.

NOTES

1. See Chapter 3.

2. See Veatch (1981) 154–5, 174; Veatch, "Medical Codes and Oaths," in Reich 3:1427–35. Veatch (1987) ix. Veatch (2000) 135. Jonsen (2000) 8. Brennan 31.

3. Pellegrino ED. "Toward an Expanded Medical Ethics: The Hippocratic Ethic Revisited," in Veatch (2000) 41–53. In a similar vein, May says that the *Oath* articulates a covenant between physicians and their teachers and describes a mere code of conduct for treating patients. May WF. "Code, Covenant, Contract or Philanthropy," in Veatch 2000, 117–34.

4. Meier 140–54.

5. Pericles. "Funeral Oration," in Copeland and Lamm 3–11.

6. Homer. *Iliad*, XI:606–7 and *Physician:14*.

7. Though "The Ambassadorial Speech of Thessalos, son of Hippocrates,"(Smith [1990] 111–25) and "The Speech at the Altar," (Smith [1990] 109), postdate the Hippocratic time, they purport to describe events of the Hippocratic time. Jouanna (14–5, 35–6) notes the late date but accepts the legitimacy of the ideas expressed in these documents.

8. Jouanna 31–3 and Smith (1950) 3–4.

9. Little is known about this office. It may have been a form of civic certification of the competence of a physician. It could have been an effort to assure that a physician was available for local citizens to hire. See Cohn-Haft L. The public physician of ancient Greece. Smith College Studies in Hist 1956;42:1–91. Jouanna 77–8.

10. Churchill reviews the notion of justice in relation to the issue of universal access to health care (Churchill).

11. I accept von Staden's later translation in part because it fits with the discussion of *diké* in MacIntyre. (1984, 134, 141) The older translations of the *Oath* are (alternative to justice is in italics): I will use my power to help the sick to the best of my ability and judgment; I will *abstain from harming or wronging any man by it....* Whenever I go into a house, I will go to help the sick and *never with the intention of doing harm*

or injury (Hippocrates [1950], p 67). Jones renders these passages as follows: I will use treatment to help the sick according to my ability and judgment; but *never with a view to injury and wrongdoing.* . . . Into whatsoever house I enter, I will enter to help the sick and I will abstain from all *intentional wrongdoing and harm*, especially from abusing the bodies of man or woman, bond or free. (Loeb I, p. 299–301).

12. Sealey 100–5, 138–42.

13. Sophocles. *Oedipus the King 957–62.*

14. Sophocles. *Antigone 499–508.*

15. Hurwitz MS. "Justice and the Metaphor of Medicine in Early Greek Thought," In Irani and Silver, 69–73.

16. MacIntyre (1988) 12–103.

17. Euripides. *Ion 252–4.*

18. Pericles. Op. cit. 4.

19. There are many places to obtain these data. The Centers for Disease Control, www.cdc.gov/nchs, is one authoritative source. The United States Census bureau is another, www.census.gov/hhes.

20. The World Health Organization. World Health Report 2000: "Health Systems: Improving Performance" http://www.who.int/whr/2000/en/report.htm

21. Starr P. What Happened to Health Care Reform? Amer Prospect 1995;20(Winter):20–31.

22. Council on Ethical and Judicial Affairs, American Medical Association. Opinions 9.065 and 2.095. 1999.

23. Plato wrote that a physician's excellence was not measured by how rich he became. The point of this text, however, is that the objective of medicine is healing. It is not a call for self-sacrificing free care. Plato. *Republic I:341c–346v.*

24. Euripides. *Electra 426–8, 1122–29.*

25. Aristophanes. *Plutus 407–8.*

26. Walzer 69–71. A full discussion of the literature on this is in Edwards ML. "Physical Disability in the Ancient World. Ph.D. diss., University of Minnesota, 1995, 44–73. Lysias 24, *On the Refusal of a Pension*, is a Greek text containing the (possibly rhetorical) defense of a person accused of unjustly seeking the disability allowance. It dates from about the time when the *Oath* was written. Athenian Constitution 49.4 describes the pension system.

27. *Regimen III:69.* Plato. *Republic 3.406 d–e.*

28. Kudlien F. Medicine as a "Liberal Art" and the question of the physician's income. J Hist Med 1976;31:448–59. See *Precepts IV, VI.*

29. Miles SH. What are we teaching about indigent patients? JAMA 1992;268; 2561–2.

30. Anonymous. The role of the physician and the medical profession in the prevention of international torture and in the treatment of its survivors. Ann Intern Med 1995;122:607–13.

31. Anonymous. Chemical and biological weaponry and war. Ann Intern Med 1969;71:204–8. Christopher GW, Cieslak TJ, Pavlin JA, Eitzen EM. Biological warfare. A historical perspective. JAMA 1997;278:412–7. Gellert GA. Global health interdependence and the international physicians' movement. JAMA 1990;264:610–3. Forrow L, Sidel VW. Medicine and nuclear war: from Hiroshima to mutual assured destruction to abolition 2000. JAMA 1998;280:456–61. Morin K, Miles SH for the American College of Physicians. Economic Sanctions and Professional Ethics. Ann Intern Med 2000;132:158–61.

32. Mann JM. Medicine and public health, ethics, and human rights, Hastings Cent Rep 1997;27(3):6–13. Bryant JH, Khan KS, Hyder AA. Ethics, equity and renewal of WHO's health-for-all strategy. World Health Forum 1997;18:107–15 (see also discussion, 116–60). See also Cambridge Quarterly 2001;10(3) for a lengthy symposium on bioethics and human rights.

33. Anonymous. World Medical Association Declaration of Helsinki: ethical principles for medical research involving human subjects. JAMA. 2000;284:3043–5; Tollman SM, Bastian H, Doll R, et al. What are the effects of the fifth revision of the Declaration of Helsinki? BMJ 2001;323(7326):1417–23. Shapiro HT, Meslin EM. Ethical issues in the design and conduct of clinical trials in developing countries. N Engl J Med 2001;345:139–42.

6

DEADLY DRUGS

I WILL NOT GIVE A DRUG THAT IS DEADLY TO ANYONE IF ASKED,
NOR WILL I SUGGEST THE WAY TO SUCH A COUNSEL.

It is a jarring idea: physicians' giving deadly drugs. Why would this issue be important enough to the ancient Greeks to merit a passage in the *Oath?* Diverse reasons have been offered. Medical ethicists tend to read this passage as a disavowal of medical euthanasia. One scholar believes that it referred to killing people during medical research. It is often cited as the historical precedent by which a physician disavowed collaborating with executions. Others say that it referred to physicians who used their medical skills to murder. Euthanasia, vivisection, execution, or murder: it is important to try to clarify the rationale for this passage in order to understand its value to the contentious debates of our time.

DEADLY DRUGS FOR EUTHANASIA?

Medical ethicists customarily interpret "I will not give a drug that is deadly," as an ancient medical disavowal of euthanasia or physician-assisted suicide.[1] For example, the National Catholic Bioethics Center has rewritten this passage to read: "I will neither prescribe nor administer a lethal dose of medicine to any patient even if asked, nor counsel any such thing nor perform act or omission with direct intent deliberately to end a human life."[2] This rendition specifies that the indefinite person referred to in authoritative translations of the *Oath* is a "patient" and it broadens the vow to encompass "omissions that are intended to end a human life." This restatement recruits the *Oath* as a precedent in support of a particular position in the modern debate about medical euthanasia and forgoing life-sustaining treatment. In fact, the history of the euthanasia debate and descriptions of the care of dying persons in ancient Greece make it unlikely that "I will not give a drug that is deadly" refers to anything like our concepts of physician-assisted suicide, voluntary or nonvoluntary euthanasia, or discontinuing life-sustaining treatment.[3]

The Greek discussion of assisted suicide or euthanasia seems to have been insufficiently developed to engender such a powerful answering taboo. Though Greek drama described characters killing themselves, phrases for *suicide* did not appear in the Greek language until after long after the *Oath* was written.[4] Even then, such phrases referred to accepting a heroic death for others or killing oneself out of shame, rather than choosing death as a way to end suffering caused by disease. Plato says that Socrates, a contemporary of Hippocrates, argued that physicians should not provide continuous, aggressive treatment to sustain the life of an incurably ill person who is "incapable of living in the established round and order of life . . . of no use either to himself or to the state."[5] Socrates' speculative proposal, however, is conceptually closer to the idea that physicians should withhold futile treatments, or triage irreversibly disabled persons away from medical care, than it is to using poison, like hemlock, for euthanasia.

The Hemlock Society has made that deadly plant and Socrates' rational choice for death rather than exile into symbols for legalizing euthanasia. The Greek medical treatises do not describe using hemlock to induce a patient's death even though the poisonous properties of the plant were well known at the time the medical books were written. Socrates died in 399 BCE, about the time the *Oath* was written. In 320 BCE, Theophrastus, the author of a compendium of biologically active plants, wrote that Thrasyas of the Greek city of Mantineia had discovered "a plant which produces an easy and painless end; he used the juices of hemlock poppy. . . . For the effect of this compound there is absolutely no cure . . . death is made swift and easy."[6] Theophrastus does not describe who used hemlock, nor for what purpose. He is also known for uncritically including folktales in his compendiums of herbal medicines.[7] Hemlock was poison, but there is no evidence that physicians used it for euthanasia.

The Greek-derived word *euthanasia* (literally: "good death") was not coined until 280 BCE, about a century after the *Oath* was written. This new word did not refer to assisting death; it referred to a natural death without agony: "Of those things that a man [human] prays for from the gods, nothing is better to meet with than an easy (happy) death."[8] *Euthanasia* continued to simply mean a peaceful dying until 1869, when the historian William Lecky gave the word its present meaning of intentionally ending life in order to end suffering from disease.[9] The ancient Greek physician knew the suffering that went with disease.

Greek clinical notes on the psychology of severe illness depicted the desire to end one's life as a sign of delirium or depression and not as a rational choice to die.[10] Depression was correctly seen as a bad prognostic sign: "[A]n over-sad countenance bodes ill."[11] "Timochareus' male servant, after what appeared melancholic affection [during the epidemic], died."[12] "For trembling to come on in patients that are out of their wits with melancholy is a malignant sign."[13] Morbid dreams, for example, dreaming of dead people, "naked or clothed in black, or not clean, or taking something or bringing something out the house, the sign is unfavorable as it indicates disease."[14] Such distressing dreams merited distinctive treatments (emetics, rest, comic diversions, a light diet, and walks). These recommendations were among the earliest proposals for palliative care of the suffering caused by disease. Ancient Greek medical texts correctly described delirium as an ominous prognostic sign. For example, *Prognostic III* records that in the case of pneumonia, grinding the teeth, "accompanied by delirium, . . . is a very deadly sign indeed."[15] The very old treatise *Epidemics III* reports: "In Thasos, the wife of Delearces, who lay sick on the plain, was seized after a grief with an acute fever with shivering. From the beginning she would wrap herself up, and throughout, without speaking a word, she would fumble, pluck, scratch, pick hairs, weep and then laugh, but she did not sleep. . . . Nineteenth day. Much wandering followed by return of reason; silent. . . . Twenty-first day. Death."[16] The astute interpretation of the mental status of serious illness as a delirium, rather than as rational or holy thoughts,[17] undercuts the foundation for interpreting a wish for death or a patient's refusal of treatment or food as an authentic desire.

People with delirium, depression, or mortal illness often refuse treatment, food, or water. The ancient Greek physicians noted this phenomenon but did not see it as indicative of a rational desire to die. The author of *Diseases* says that persons with phrenitis, "Being deranged, they do not accept anything worth mentioning that is administered to them and as time passes, they waste away and become emaciated as a result of their fever and of the fact that nothing is entering their body. . . . Finally everything becomes cold and the person dies."[18] *Epidemics I* describes a twenty-year-old man who was "attacked by fever . . . thirst; tongue dry . . . no urine . . . took no drink" until he slipped into a coma and died.[19] In these cases, anorexia was seen as integral to a lethal disease rather than as a willful desire to die. There is nothing to suggest that the acquiescence of the physician to this process was analogous to giving a deadly drug.[20]

Greek physicians advised treating persons who were suicidal or who had self-inflicted wounds. *Epidemic V* reported, "The woman who cut her throat: she choked. She was later given much purgative medicine. . . ."[21] *Places in Man* offered this advice, "To those who are troubled and ill and want to hang themselves, give mandrake root to drink in the morning, an amount less than would make them delirious."[22] Unlike the discussions of abortion by midwives, the medical treatises do not describe physicians, other healers, or lay people helping sick people commit suicide.[23]

Though there is no evidence that Greek physicians assisted suicide or practiced euthanasia, they seem to have expressed contradictory ideas about treating those who were terminally ill. Some texts argued in favor of treating mortally ill people; others said that attempting to cure those who are dying did not properly belong to medicine. The ancient Greek physicians recognized that they must not engage in cultic practices or conceit that implied that medicine could vanquish death. Asclepius was punished for raising the dead. As the author of *The Art*, one of the most respected Greek medical works, writes:

> I would define medicine as the complete removal of the distress of the sick, the alleviation of the more violent diseases, and the refusal to undertake to cure cases in which the disease has already won the mastery, knowing that everything is not possible to medicine. . . . A man who thinks that a science can perform what is outside its province, or that nature can accomplish unnatural things is guilty of ignorance more akin to madness than to lack of learning.[24]

With such a view, it is not surprising that some material suggested that it was proper to withhold treatment that merely prolongs dying. For example, one of the *Aphorisms* says: "It is better not to treat those who have internal cancers since if not treated, they die quickly: but if treated they last a long time."[25] Some medical ethicists incorrectly cite such material as proof that Greek physicians did not believe in treating incurably ill persons.

In fact, Greek physicians described caring for many hopelessly ill persons.[26] Sixty percent of the case reports ended in death. Some doctors cared for dying patients for long periods. *Epidemics III*, one of the oldest medical works, describes "the man from Pharos who lay beyond the Temple of Artemis"; he developed a fever, became delirious on the seventeenth day, and was intermittently awake and mostly comatose until he died on the 120th day, with the physician making frequent medical notes during this four months.[27] The many case records of the care of dying persons describe a profession that treated incurably ill patients, provided that the dire prognosis was disclosed. (See Chapter 10 on disclosing prognoses.) For example, the authors of *Joints* and *Fractures* recommend partial, palliative treatment of fractures where the bones have penetrated the flesh to be exposed to the air.[28] The author of *Internal Affections* recommends conventional treatment even for people with indolent, terminal illnesses: "Another consumption: . . . death from this disease usually occurs in three years. You must treat with the same things that you gave to the preceding patient. This disease continues in most patients up to three years but still they die; for it is severe."[29] Do the various statements on treating incurably ill patients represent a division in the ancient medical community or simply underscore our difficulty understanding a different medical culture that could unify these seemingly contradictory recommendations?

Contemporary physicians have a medical model that understands how to treat pain even without treating the underlying disease. Morphine, for example, alleviates the pain of bone cancer without treating the cancer itself. In contrast, Greek medicine had a holistic understanding that integrated the cause and symptoms of a disease in a way that also fused curative and palliative remedies. As the ancient author of *Places in Man* elegantly wrote:

> There is no beginning in the body; but everything is alike beginning and end. For when a circle has been drawn, its beginning is not to be found. And the beginning of ailments comes from the entire body alike. . . . Each part of the body at once transmits illness one to the other. . . . Thus, it is best to treat parts which are ill by the situations which bring about the illness. For in this way one would best remedy the beginning of the illness. The body is homogenous . . .

and if you like to take the smallest part of the body and injure it, the whole body will feel the injury. . . . For this reason the body feels pain or pleasure from its smallest constituent because all parts exist in the smallest part and these refer everything to each of their own related parts, and register everything.[30]

With such a view, treating a disease eased pain and treating pain alleviated the disease.

In addition to benefiting incurably ill persons, the Greek physicians valued such care for what they could learn as well. The author of *Joints* explicitly stated the case for attending to people with incurable diseases in order to advance medical science.

Why, forsooth, trouble one's mind further about cases that have become incurable? This is far from the right attitude. The investigation of these matters too belongs to the same science; it is impossible to separate them from one another. In curable cases, we must contrive ways to prevent their becoming incurable, studying the best means for hindering their advance to incurability; while one must study incurable cases so as to avoid doing harm by useless efforts.[31]

Attempting to cure, palliating suffering, and advancing the science: these three goals defined the engagement of Greek physicians with dying persons. If medically assisted euthanasia had been part of the care of the dying by physicians, herbalists, or midwives, it seems likely that physicians would have noted it just as abortions would have been discussed. There is no evidence that this passage spoke to an ancient debate about medical euthanasia.

DEADLY DRUGS FOR RESEARCH ON HUMANS?

Lloyd proposes that "I will not give a drug that is deadly" is a disavowal of vivisection. He cites Celsus' charge against third-century BCE anatomists Herophilius and Erasistratus, who worked at Alexandria.[32]

They laid open men whilst alive—criminals received out of prison from the kings—and whilst these were still breathing, observed parts which beforehand nature had concealed, their position, color, shape, size, arrangement, hardness, softness, smoothness, relation, processes and depressions of each and whether any part is inserted into another or received into another.[33]

There are several reasons to reject Lloyd's hypothesis. First, as Edelstein points out, this interpretation of "I will not give a deadly drug" is chronologically untenable because ancient Greek physicians carefully recorded observations of deep tissues that had been exposed by trauma, disease or surgery, but did not perform nontherapeutic dissection or autopsies.[34] Furthermore, Herophilius and Erasistratus lived a century after the *Oath* was written and worked in the medical culture of Alexandria. Many scholars doubt the veracity of the charge against Herophilius and Erasistratus and believe that it arose long after their deaths and was motivated by jealously among anatomists. Second, Greek physicians believed that a person who touched a corpse was polluted.[35] Vivisection would have conflicted with the portion of the *Oath* in which the physician vows to remain free of pollution: "in a pure and holy way I will guard my life and my [professional work]." Third, Athens' laws had no exemption for vivisection. At best, Celsus' condemnation reflects a moral concern of the first century CE, 500 years after the *Oath* was written. It is improbable that "I will not give a drug that is deadly" refers to vivisection.

PHYSICIANS AS EXECUTIONERS?

Ancient Greece practiced capital punishment. The ancient Greek record is silent on whether physicians were asked to participate in executions or offer technical advice to make execution more effective or humane. The physician as executioner does not appear to have been an issue for public discussion and for that reason seems unlikely to have inspired the *Oath's* words on "deadly drugs."

Physician engagement in making executions more humane is best dated to 1789, when the French physician-legislator, Joseph-Ignace Guillotin, successfully promoted a law against torture that required that all executions be carried out by means of a "machine that beheads painlessly." Until then, only the elite were afforded the courtesy of such a painless "final exit." Some physicians in the United States have assisted with execution by lethal injection by selected drugs or adjusting dosages according to a person's medical condition. Though medical associations condemn such practices, they do not seem to want physicians to be accountable to such disavowals. [36]

PHYSICIANS AS MURDERERS?

I agree with Littré that "I will not give a drug that is deadly" addresses the fear that physicians would collaborate with murder by poisoning.[37] Murder was common in the ancient world, especially at the time the *Oath* was written, during the turmoil after the defeat of Athens by Sparta in 405 BCE. Murder eliminated kings, successors, competitors, and municipal figures. A wealthy family, for example, overthrew Hippias, dictator of Athens in 510 BCE after his brother was assassinated. In 460 BCE, after interfering with a Greek Council, Phialtes was assassinated. In 413 BCE, Archelaus used assassination to become king of Macedon. In 336 BCE, Phillip of Macedon was assassinated, probably at the behest of his wife, the mother of Alexander the Great. Each succeeding assassination set the stage for revenge murders or further killings to regain power lost through the previous murder. Countless murders for gain went unrecorded. Physicians were bound by oaths requiring them to assist their city-state. They were personally connected to military or civil leaders or wealthy patrons. Moral conflicts arising from duty to the state were keenly felt, widely discussed, and well documented.[38] As the *Oath* was being written, the Athenian economy was collapsing, fewer city-physicians were being hired, and physicians were under economic pressure.[39] In such a world, physicians had the skills for poisoning, trusted access, and would have been vulnerable to coercion or temptation to join in homicidal schemes.

Fear of the physician-poisoner may be traced very close to the time of the *Oath*. In 345 BCE, Plato wrote that a physician who administers a poison with the intention of causing death should be executed, as such deeds are acts of terror.[40] Plato's depiction of the physician who poisons is a discussion of skilled and secret assassin and bears no similarity to compassionate medical euthanasia or physician-assisted suicide. Edelstein asserted that ancient physicians routinely killed patients but his sources describe malevolent homicides rather than medically assisted death to end suffering. Most of his accounts come from Roman and Christian societies centuries after the *Oath* was written.[41] For example, Pliny (23–79 CE) quotes Cato, a xenophobic Roman, as saying that Greek physicians were barbarians who were preoccupied with death, expert in poison, and potential assassins.[42] Tacitus tells how are physician, Gaius Stertinius Xenophon, murdered the Roman emperor Claudius in 54 CE. Claudius's wife, Agrippina, wanted to ensure that the empire passed to her son by a previous marriage, Nero. She asked a convicted poisoner, Locusta, about poison mushrooms. The tale, though late, is representative of the stories of physicians' administering deadly drugs that are found in the ancient literature.

> . . . the poison was sprinkled on a particularly succulent mushroom. But because Claudius was torpid or drunk, its effect was not at first apparent. An evacuation of the bowels seemed to save him. Agrippina was horrified. . . . She had already secured the complicity of Xenophon; and now she called him in. . . . While pretending to help Claudius to vomit, he put a feather dipped in a quick poison down his throat. Xenophon knew that major crimes, though hazardous to undertake are profitable to achieve.[43]

Scholars believe that much of this literature is a genre of fiction or satire[44] somewhat akin to modern medical horror novels. Fictional or not, the ancient physician with the deadly drug came as an assassin and not as a friend.

There is another piece of evidence that this passage refers to the crime of murder rather than the misplaced compassion of euthanasia. "I will not give a drug that is deadly" follows the words "from injustice I will keep them" and thus seems to speak of the doctor's refusing to act at the behest of others who would commit an injustice in the public world. If this vow had been situated after "Into the houses I enter . . . while being far from all voluntary and destructive injustice," it seems more probable that it would have been a vow to refrain from using poison to end suffering during a clinical relationship. The physician-assassin damaged the trustworthiness of the entire profession, and the *Oath's* simple vow spoke to this fear.

There are still physicians who exploit their access to medical tools to commit murder.[45] Such crimes are probably the closest descendents of the transgressions alluded to by this passage. In addition to criminal sanctions, such physicians are expelled from the practice of medicine, though in truth they exile themselves. The *Oath* did not anticipate the scale of medical homicide that was practiced by Nazi physicians who designed and supervised mass executions and genocide and who engaged in vivisection.[46] That large-scale collaboration between the medical profession and a genocidal government in crimes against humanity seems to call for history's judgment rather than some a simple courtroom proceeding. The *Oath* addresses history's judgment on medicine in its closing passage.

                                    *   *   *

CASE 6.1 "Dr. Miles, I want you to give me a medicine so that I can end my life." I had first met Mary Hansen for a physical examination only a week earlier. She was ostensibly returning for a routine follow-up to review the laboratory results and adjust her medications. She was 85 and without relatives. She lived in a Lutheran retirement community that had an attached nursing home and clinic. The first time I saw her, my impression was of gray hair, a set, pale face, a woman who was polite, dignified, and reserved. She had osteoporosis of the spine and arthritis of both hips, painful conditions for which a specialist had prescribed an anti-inflammatory drug. She walked with a labored stoop. She had withdrawn from her friends.

I was taken aback by this request from a person whom I had known for such a brief time. My reply went something like this: "I am sorry you feel this way. I cannot help you by giving you drugs to end your life. But tell me why you feel that way, then give me six weeks to see if I can make you feel the way you want to feel." She talked about being in pain and being disabled and no longer seeing her friends. I stopped the anti-inflammatory drug and prescribed regular doses of a narcotic and an antidepressant. One out of three people with chronic disease is depressed; treatment for depression lifts their mood and decreases disability. We spoke on the telephone as she increased the dose of the narcotic.

I saw Ms. Hansen in the clinic a week after she started taking the narcotics. Her gait was less painful. Two weeks later, her mood seemed better, although I did not know if this was due to the narcotic or to the antidepressant. Three weeks after her request to die, she walked into the exam room with her hair freshly tinted blue—a fashion in her community and evidence that she had visited the beauty salon in the basement. I suggested that she start going to the dining room instead of eating alone in her apartment. She did so and took up socializing again with her old friends.

She never repeated her request for assistance with suicide. Seven months after our initial meeting, she suffered a major stroke that left her paralyzed, unable to speak, and barely conscious. In compliance with her Living Will, I did not use life support or a feeding tube. She died within a week.

A couple of weeks after her death, a lacquered wood box and a letter arrived at the clinic. The box contained ashes. The note in Mary's own hand said, "Dear Dr. Miles, I want to thank you for being my doctor. I have given all my belongings to others who could use them. This is what is left. I am giving a third to you, a third to my visiting nurse, and a third to my social worker. Mary Hansen." On the way home with this odd bequest, I remembered that ashes are acidic. As I write these words, an acid-loving, salmon-colored Spicy Lights azalea marks another spring in my garden.

What advice does "I will not give a drug that is deadly to anyone if asked, nor will I suggest the way to such a counsel," have for physicians today? Many people believe that this passage disavows medical euthanasia or physician-assisted suicide. Such a reading would imply a particular answer to Ms. Hansen's request for my help with her suicide. Though we may choose to read this meaning into the *Oath*, I do not believe that the ancient Greeks anticipated this application. Even so, the ancient Greek medical treatises contain some advice about a person like Ms. Hansen. Those physicians would have interpreted her request for a lethal drug as a bad prognostic sign, part of the "over-sad countenance that bodes ill," rather than as a rational request to die. Physicians continued to treat mortally ill persons sometimes, as in the physician of the "man in Pharos," for a long time.

There are other similarities and differences in the care of people near the end of their lives by physicians in the United States and those of ancient Greece. Both medical cultures failed to make treating pain a primary palliative objective. But Greek physicians' understanding of disease imperfectly separated treating pain from treating the underlying disease. Though palliative treatment of pain is far better understood today, American physicians tend to undertreat pain, especially for persons in the final days of life. In Ms. Hansen's case, a specialist tried to decrease the inflammation of her arthritis (the cause of pain) rather than treating the pain itself. That approach was part of why she came to my clinic requesting drugs to end her life. Ironically, a holistic Greek approach that saw the pain and depression as an integrated syndrome might have pointed to an earlier and more effective response to her suffering before the stroke that took her life.

The stroke took Ms. Hansen's physical and cognitive abilities. She could have been sustained on life-support until she died. Greek physicians lacked both technology and an ethic for prolonging dying.[47] When confronted with an incurably ill, gravely disabled, and dying patient, it appears that Greek physicians would have recognized a duty to defer to the mastery of death. I did not insert a feeding tube to sustain Ms. Hansen's life. The idea of not employing a feeding tube for a mortally ill person who was not taking fluid was not technologically envisioned in the ancient Greece. Yet, even though the Greek physicians recommended special diets and fluids to nourish severely ill persons,[48] they did not describe force-feeding patients who would not take food or fluid. The lack of interest or ability to take food and fluids was described as intrinsic to mortal illness. For example, *Epidemics III* describes a case: "In Thasos the Parian who lay sick beyond the temple of Artemis was seized with acute fever. . . . Thirst. . . . Aversion to food. . . . He took little bits of food, and that of an unsuitable sort. . . . Death."[49] The naturalism of this observation does not seem coarse; it seems intimate—the physician was caring for this man as he died.

NOTES

1. Beauchamp and Childress 226. May 92. Thomasma and Pellegrino 120. Kass 234. Kamisar Y. "Some Non-religious View Against Proposed 'Mercy Killing Legislation,'" in Horan and Mall 421. Mall D. "Death and the Rhetoric of Unknowing" in Horan and Mall 650. Anagnostopoulos G. "Euthanasia and the Physician's Role: Reflections on Some Views in the Ancient Greek Tradition," in Kuczewski and Polansky 251–90. Kass LR. "'I will give no deadly drug': Why doctors must not kill," in Thomasma and Kushner, 239–45. Verhey A. The doctor's oath—And a Christian swearing it. Linacre Quarterly 1984;51(2):139–58. The view that physicians' opposition to performing euthanasia is based on the Hippocratic Oath is also asserted by the American Medical Association (Anonymous. Decisions Near the End of Life. JAMA 1992; 267: 2229–233) and the American College of Physicians—American Society of Internal Medicine (Snyder L, Sulmasy DP, for the Ethics and Human Rights Committee. Ann Intern Med 2001;135:209–16). Veatch acknowledges the ambiguity and debate about this passage but does not explain why he concludes that it refers to euthanasia or assisted suicide (Veatch RM. "Medical Codes and Oaths: Ethical Analysis," in Reich 1431). Jonsen seems equally open to the idea that the passage refers to murder or assassination (Jonsen [2000] 4 and [1998] 262).

2. Value of Life Committee. "The 1995 Restatement of the Oath of Hippocrates, circa 400 BC." National Catholic Bioethics Center, Boston, MA 02135 (available at www.ncbcenter.org).

3. For discussion of the modern debate about assisted suicide see: Emanuel EJ, Fairclough DL, Emanuel LL. Attitudes and desires related to euthanasia and physician-assisted suicide among terminally ill patients and their caregivers. JAMA 2000; 284:2460–8. Sullivan AD, Hedberg K, Fleming DW. Legalized physician-assisted suicide in Oregon—the second year. N Engl J Med 2000;342:598–604. Snyder L, Sulmasy DP for the Ethics and Human Rights Committee, American College of Physicians—American Society of Internal Medicine. Ann Int Med 2001;135:209–16. I oppose legalizing physician-assisted suicide, for example, in "Assisted suicide and the profession's gyrocompass." Hastings Cent Rep 1995;25(3):17–9.

4. Daube D. The linguistics of suicide. Philosophy & Public Affairs 1972;1:387–437. Hastings XII: 26–31) looks at the phrasing and means of suicide in ancient Greece.

Sophocles, for example, describes the suicides of Jocasta (wife and mother of Oedipus) and the shamed soldier and protagonist Ajax. These suicides were engendered by shame, not illness. Edelstein argues that poison was the most common means of suicide in ancient Greece but his cited examples date to hundreds of years after the *Oath* (Edelstein, "The Hippocratic Oath: Text, Translation, and Interpretation," in Temkin and Temkin 11–13). He cites accounts in *Metamorphosis* X:9–10 (170 CE), *Golden Ass* X:9 (170 CE) *Vita Hadriani* XXIV:13 (4th CE), *Libanius Progymnasia* 8 (4th CE), *Ephesian Tale* (3rd CE).

    5. Plato. *Republic III, 405a-410a*

    6. Theophrastus. IX,16

    7. Lloyd (1983) 120–135.

    8. I am indebted to Gerald Erickson, retired professor of Classical and Near Eastern Studies at the University of Minnesota, for this translation. This is found in an anthology of fragments of ancient writings that was compiled in the fifth century CE by Stobareus. The quote is from a lost comedy, *Myrmex (The Ant)*, by Posidippus Comicus. (*Comicorum Atticorum Fragmenta*. Ed. T Kock, Vol. 111. Paris: B.G. Teuberi, 1888.)

    9. Lecky WEH. "History of European Morals" (1869) I:ix;223 described euthanasia as "an abridgement of the pangs of disease." Citation from Compact Oxford English Dictionary (2nd ed.), Oxford: Clarenden Press, 1991. See also Cooper JM. "Greek Philosophers on Euthanasia and Suicide," in Brody 9–38; and Carrick 58.

    10. Examples of astute comments on mental illness and chronic disease are at: *Aphorisms* II:vi; *Aphorisms* VI:xxiii; *Epidemics* 2.6:1; *Epidemics* 5:85; *Epidemics* 7:89. Lloyd also comments on Greek psychiatry (Lloyd [1987] 21–9).

    11. *Prorrhetic* I:49. See also *Epidemics* 6.2:17 and *Epidemics* 5:84.

    12. *Epidemics* 5:87.

    13. *Prorrhetic* I:14. There are many other cases of depression: for example, see *Prorrhetic* I:44, 123; *Epidemics III*: case 6, 2, 11.

    14. *Dreams* XCII. See also *Dreams* LXXXVIII, LXXXIX, XC, and XCIII.

    15. *Prognostic III*. There are many other cases of delirium that are discussed in the oldest of the *Aphorisms* 6:LIII, 7:V, XIV, XXIV; *Disease* II:65; *Epidemics* I, III, V, VII; *Prorrhetic* I:8, 19, 26, 49; *On Fractures* xi.

    16. *Epidemics III; sixteen cases: xv.*

    17. The physicians' clinical view of the significance of dreams as symptoms was unlike the view held by temple healers, who saw dreams as a form of intuitive divination by lay people (Lloyd [1987] 30–7). Temple healers and physicians both discerningly listened to dreams, hallucinations, and delusions, and used them in their diagnostic and prognostic craft even though they sharply differed on the divine vs. natural grounding of such phenomena. Langhoff's assertion (247) that such natural

divination by patients had no counterpart in medical prognosis is somewhat extreme. A more nuanced discussion is in Oberhelman SM. The diagnostic dream in ancient medical theory and practice. Bull Hist Med 1987;61:47–60.

18. *Diseases 1:34*. See also: *Epidemics I (fourteen cases) Case II*; *Epidemics III (Case IX)*; *Epidemics III (Sixteen cases) Case II, Case XVI*; *Diseases I:34*; *Epidemics III (sixteen cases) Case I*.

19. *Epidemics I (fourteen cases) Case II*. See also: *Epidemics III (Case IX)*, *Epidemics III (sixteen cases) Case II, Case XVI*, and *Diseases I:34*.

20. This is potential problem in the National Catholic Bioethics Center restatement of the Hippocratic Oath, which interprets giving a deadly drug as also encompassing any "omission with direct intent deliberately to end a human life." Attending to a patient who is known to not take food when one knows that food could extend life may be such an omission.

21. *Epidemics 5:33*. *Epidemics 6.8:20* may describe another suicide attempt.

22. *Places in Man 39* (Hippocrates [1998]).

23. Nicholson, op cit.

24. *The Art 1:8* (Trans from Chadwick who calls it *"The Science of Medicine"*).

25. *Aphorisms 6:38* (Hippocrates [1950]).

26. Prioreschi P. Did the Hippocratic physician treat hopeless cases? Gesnerus 1992;49:341–350.

27. *Epidemics III (sixteen cases) Case I*.

28. *Joints LXIII–LXVI, Fractures XXXV–VI*. This may account for Jouanna's observation about the inattention of Hippocratic physicians to pain control, other than to minimizing the additional pain caused by their procedures (Jouanna 127–8, 326).

29. *Internal Affections 11*.

30. *Places in Man 1* (Hippocrates 1998).

31. *On Joints LVIII*.

32. Lloyd (1977) 356, 357, 359, 360, 413. Lloyd also notes an account of Mithridates who, in the first century CE, poisoned prisoners to test antidotes to protect himself from assassination.

33. Celsus. *De Medicine, Proemium to Book I, 23*.

34. Edelstein L. "The History of Anatomy in Antiquity," in Temkin and Temkin, 247–302. Lloyd cited Edelstein on this point but did not respond to this critique. See also Lloyd (1991) 167–93 and Drabkin IE. On medical education in Greece and Rome. Bull Hist Med 1944;15:333–51. The Hippocratic treatise *On the Heart* contains a superb description of the internal anatomy of the heart, but it dates from the second century BCE, centuries after the *Oath* was written.

35. von Staden H. The discovery of the body: Human dissection and its cultural contexts in ancient Greece. Yale J Biol Med 1992;223–41.

36. A correctional health care physician, Dr. Kim Thorburn, sued California to prevent physicians from assisting in capital punishment. She argued that the state law of medical practice barred physicians from engaging in "unprofessional conduct." Though the California Medical Association, the American Medical Association, the American College of Physicians, and two societies of correctional health professionals officially hold that physicians may not assist in executions, those societies were reluctant to have collaboration with executions become an area for sanctions against physicians. Accordingly, they declined to join the lawsuit and it failed. Thorburn v. Department of Corrections (1998) 66 Cal. App. 4th 1284, 1290, fn. 6 [78 Cal. Rptr. 2d 584] and Brief of Medical Ethics Scholars as Amicus Curiae in support of Plaintiff-Appellants (Thorburn v Department of Corrections) at http://www.bumc.bu.edu/ www/sph/lw/pvl/amicus.html.

37. Littré Vol IV:624.

38. MacIntyre (1988) 42–68.

39. Aristophanes. *Plutus 407–8.*

40. Plato. *Laws 933.*

41. See Edelstein, above, and Kudlien F. Medical ethics and popular ethics in Greece and Rome. Clio Med 1970;5:91–121. Ratzan RM, Ferngran GB. A Greek progymasma on the physician-poisoner. J Hist Med Allied Sci 1993;48:157–70. Jonsen apparently conducted a similarly fruitless search. "Apart from occasional references to assisted death, as when Roman physician Scribonius Largus condemns physicians who take life, the medical literature of antiquity ignores the subject." (Jonsen [1998] 262).

42. Kudlien F. Medical ethics and popular ethics in Greece and Rome. Clio Med 1970;5:91–121.

43. Tacitus 279–82.

44. These stories can be found in Amundsen DW. Romanticizing the ancient medical profession: The characterization of the physician in the Greco-Roman novel. Bull Hist Med, 1974;48:320–37. Gourevitch D. Suicide among the sick in classical antiquity. Bull Hist Med 1969:43:501–18. Amundsen DW. The liability of the physician in classical Greek legal theory and practice. J Hist Med Allied Sci 1977;32:172–204.

45. Iserson.

46. Lifton. Proctor.

47. Amundsen DW. The physician's obligation to prolong life: A medical duty without classical roots. Hastings Cent Rep 1978(Aug):23–30.

48. *Affections 10, 18, 19,2539, 43–60* compiles many medical diets. *Epidemics I XIX, and (fourteen cases) Case VI* describe severely ill patients who were notably able to eat.

49. *Epidemics III (sixteen cases) Case I.*

7

ABORTION

AND LIKEWISE I WILL NOT GIVE A WOMAN A DESTRUCTIVE PESSARY.

Opponents of medical abortion cite this passage from the *Oath* as evidence that medical ethics has disavowed abortion since the inception of the profession.[1] Excepting Jonsen, contemporary bioethicists largely accept an interpretation of the *Oath* that opposes abortions.[2] Verhey claims that the *Oath* marks an ethical turning point in medicine: "For centuries before the *Oath*, ancient physicians had provided poison for those whom they could not heal, had counted abortifacents among the tools of their trade, and had been disposed to the use of the knife instead of the less invasive use of dietetics and pharmacology."[3] The National Catholic Bioethics Center's "Restatement of the Oath of Hippocrates, circa 400 B.C." amends these words to read: "I will maintain the utmost respect for every human life from fertilization to natural death and reject abortion that deliberately takes a unique human life."[4] The medical ethics of abortion in ancient Greece and the meaning of this passage from the *Oath* are not so clear.

An attempt to understand what this passage meant in ancient Greece, and thus its potential extrapolation to our time, must address several puzzles. First, though Greek society saw fertility and pregnancy as healthy and socially desirable, abortion was legal and frequently described. Second, the passage refers only to "destructive pessaries" despite the fact that Greeks used a variety of abortive methods. Third, cultural values changed enormously after the *Oath* was written, and the position that killing a fetus morally resembled killing a person does not seem to have been articulated until after the *Oath* was written. These apparent paradoxes can be better understood, and perhaps partly resolved, by reviewing what the ancient medical works say about the destructive pessary, the status of women in gynecology, the moral status of the fetus, and finally, how this portion of the *Oath* was received and transformed by history.

THE DESTRUCTIVE PESSARY

Vaginal pessaries were commonly used in ancient Greece. These were wool tampons soaked in a variety of substances, including: opium poppies, bitter almond oil, boiled honey, sea onion, ox marrow, goose fat, rose oil, thapsia root, myrtle, coriander, cumin, marjoram, bacchar (an aromatic root), perfumes, emetics, or other substances.[5] The following is a typical account of the use of a therapeutic pessary:

> The wife of Epicrates, who lay sick near the statue of the city founder, when near her delivery was seized with severe rigor without, it was said, becoming warm and the same symptoms occurred the following day. On the third day, she gave birth to a daughter and the delivery was in every respect normal. On the second day after the delivery, she was seized with acute fever, pain at the stomach and in the genitals. A pessary relieved these symptoms. . . .[6]

Pessaries appear to have been a second-line treatment in that they were known to have the risk of abrading or lacerating the vagina and thereby causing infections. For example, "If the uterus is not affected by [vapor baths, mild drugs, diet therapy], one must purge it by means of non-biting drugs administered as pessaries. But always administer vapor baths before the purgatives."[7] The *Oath's* "destructive pessary" is believed to be one that induced an abortion.

Abortion was legal in ancient Greece. Greek medical texts described many women after spontaneous and induced abortions.[8] The ancient accounts often did not distinguish between induced and spontaneous abortions (miscarriages).[9] Sometimes the woman did not tell the physician how the abortion came to be.

For example: "Simus' wife had an abortion on the thirtieth day, [whether] from drinking something, or spontaneously."[10] In the following discussion from *Diseases in Women*, the physician described abortion as a secret practice that took place among women. He notes that secrecy makes it difficult to determine whether a subsequent inflammation of the uterus is caused by the trauma of miscarrying a large fetus, or by a harsh pessary, or by both.

> Suppose after an abortion a woman receives a serious lesion or that she causes ulcerations in her uterus with harsh pessaries (such as women produce in treating themselves and others), and her fetus is destroyed and the women herself is not cleansed, but her uterus becomes very inflamed and closes. . . .[11]

The treatises discuss how to try to treat a potential miscarriage [12] but do not describe any attempt to medically reverse an abortion that a woman had electively and deliberately induced. *On the Diseases of Women* gives detailed instructions on how to dismember a dead fetus that is retained in the uterus.[13] The overall picture that emerges seems to be one where physicians were practicing in a culture where abortion was not infrequent but where it was largely performed within a women's culture.

The risks of abortion to a woman's health were recognized and feared. One physician noted, "Abortions are more dangerous than births because it is impossible for an embryo to be aborted by medicine or by a potion or by food or by pessaries or in any way at all without applying force, and force is a painful thing. The risk here is that the womb will become lacerated or inflamed and this is dangerous."[14] As a result, a physician noted, women were damaging themselves with abortion "all the time."[15] It is reasonable to hypothesize that orally administered potions or destructive vaginal pessaries were actually abortive adjuvants that were intended to kill the fetus or weaken its attachment to the uterine wall. Such adjuvants would have been followed by a forceful procedure (possibly uterine kneading or the insertion of sticks or plants into the uterus) to complete the abortion. Such forceful methods are widely practiced in developing countries today. Given that pessaries were a second-line therapy because of their risks of causing infection, the specific ban on using destructive pessaries as an abortive adjuvant may reflect a clinical insight that the combined use of a foreign body in the vagina with uterine force or instrumentation unacceptably increased the feared and often-lethal infections. It seems plausible that a physician would have been held responsible for a death that was proximate in bodily location and time to the use of a destructive pessary.[16] This may explain why the passage only refers to abortion by a "destructive pessary" when oral abortifacents were known and described in medical works.[17]

WOMEN, MEN, AND GYNECOLOGY

Physicians were male. Phanostrate was a notable exception. She was a midwife and physician during the time of the Hippocratic School and was publicly celebrated as causing "pain to no one and all lamented her death."[18] The ancient Greek medical treatises describe gynecological health care; some entirely specialized on this topic.[19] These works show three forces at work that are relevant to understanding the issues raised by abortion. They depict a male perspective on women and the evolution of a comprehensive set of medical theories and treatments based on those theories. Equally importantly, they reveal the status of women as patients.

Gynecology quickly developed a comprehensive and male-centered view of the female patient. Therapeutic pessaries were not only used to treat uterine diseases (e.g., infertility,[20] postpartum infections,[21] retained placentas,[22] and amenorrhea[23]). They also were therapeutic, along with sex and marriage, in treating other conditions that were attributed to an "obstructed, disordered, or wandering" uterus (e.g., heartburn, suicidality, homicidal rage, hallucinations, depression, jaundice, sleepiness, and nasal congestion.[24]) One text went as far as to say, "As for what are called women's diseases: the womb is responsible for all such diseases."[25] Male physicians prescribed treatments for disorders of pregnancy, such as toxemia.[26] They also prescribed contraception, "If a woman does not wish to become pregnant, dissolve in water, misy as large as a bean and give it to her to drink, and for a year she will not become pregnant."[27] As the *Oath* notes, women were denied positions as medical teachers or students. Dr. Demand, a scholar of Greek medicine, says that the ascent of male obstetricians and the medicalization of pregnancy was a historic step toward greater male control over women's reproductive lives.[28]

The advent of physicians and their male view of gynecology brought this area of practice into alignment with the gender rules and roles in ancient Greece. Greece society set a high—and double—standard to safeguard the chastity of free women.[29] Though not cloistered, free women largely lived in the company of other women and their husbands or the male head of the house. New tensions arose as medicine brought men to gynecology. Here, for example, Euripides portrays a nurse speaking to her ailing mistress: "If you are sick and it is some secret sickness [an adulterous pregnancy may be fairly inferred], here are women standing at your side to help. But if your troubles may be told to men, speak, that a doctor may pronounce upon it."[30] The arrival of a male obstetrician-gynecologist posed new ethical problems for medical practice, social problems for women seeking medical care, and a challenge to the authority of male guardians of women.

Gynecological interviews or examinations were problematic under existing sexual norms. Even after the arrival of physicians, midwives or female herbalists continued to perform much of the gynecology and nursing care and assisted physicians during surgery on women.[31] Sometimes a midwife or another woman took the female patient's medical history for a male physician. Sometimes a midwife examined or performed a gynecological procedure under the supervision of a male physician.[32] Sometimes a woman examined or manipulated her own vagina or cervix according to the physician's instruction.[33] By such measures, the physical modesty of a health-care encounter could be respected; respect for the personal autonomy of a woman patient was more difficult to maintain.

Greek women were not empowered to make their own medical choices. A male guardian [kyrios] was responsible for each wife, female slave, or unmarried free-woman.[34] The guardian assumed financial responsibility, spoke for the woman in court, authorized her marriage, and distributed her estate as a dowry.[35] The guardian also safeguarded a woman's sexual chastity, authorized medical treatment, and decided whether her unwanted infant would be exposed to die.[36] Sophocles alluded to the need for such a guardian in describing Oedipus' appeal to his daughters' uncle to become their guardian as Oedipus went into exile. "Oh Creon, you are the only father they have now . . . don't let them go begging, abandoned, women without men."[37] The medical treatises reflected this culture of guardianship as they identified men by name and women as the nameless wives or daughters of named men.[38] Marriage transferred guardianship in a ceremony that often focused on childbearing, like the following:

FATHER: I give you my daughter to sow for the purpose of producing legitimate children.
GROOM: I take her.

FATHER: I also give you a dowry of three talents.
GROOM: I take it gladly.[39]

This dependence of women had profound implications for the physician–patient–guardian relationship in gynecology and can even be seen in the gynecological theories themselves.

Though women gave birth, they were considered biologically subordinate progenitors. One medical treatise claimed that a man usually determined the sex of his offspring because his boy-baby or girl-baby sperm was stronger than the "sperm" of a woman, though it concedes that sometimes the quantity of a woman's sexed seed could overwhelm a man's sperm, thereby enabling her to determine the baby's sex.[40] A more extreme view likened a uterus to a man's field (as suggested in the use of the word "sow" in the marriage ritual cited above). For example, Aeschylus quoted Apollo as saying:

> Here is the truth, I tell you—see how right I am. The woman you call the mother of the child is not the parent, just a nurse to the seed, the new-sown seed that grows and swells inside her. The man is the source of life—the one who mounts. She, like a stranger for a stranger, keeps the shoot alive. . . .[41]

The fetus belonged to the man who determined its sex and whose permission was needed to set it out to die by exposure if it was unwanted. With this gendered view of gynecological science and of the limited autonomy of women, a woman had reason to believe that a physician would disclose information about an abortion to a husband, owner, or father, and defer to the guardian's wishes. The physician was working on behalf of the guardian's authority and duties. For a male physician to perform an abortion without a guardian's consent risked fostering the charge that the physician was trespassing on the man's household or marriage, destroying what he had "sown" on his "field," or concealing the product of an illicit sexual act between the woman and the physician or another man.

An account of a physician inducing abortion illuminates the complex relationship with regard to abortion between a physician, a pregnant woman, and her guardian or owner.

> A kinswoman of mine owned a very valuable flute girl. It was important that this girl should not become pregnant and thereby lose her value. [The girl missed a

period.] She told her mistress and the story came to me. . . . I told her to jump
up and down, touching her buttocks with her heels at each leap. After she had
done this no more than seven times, there was a noise; the seed fell out . . . it
was as though someone had removed the shell from a raw egg so that the fluid
inside showed through the inner membrane. . . . In the middle of the membrane
was a small projection: it looked to me like an umbilicus. . . . From it, the membrane stretched all around the seed.[42]

In that the Greek records do not record physicians' moral transgressions, the
fact that this clinical event was recorded suggests that may have been a morally acceptable example of how to perform an abortion. The physician carefully recorded that the owner brought the patient to him and was requesting
the abortion, which the woman assented to. The fact that the owner was a relative perhaps implies a special kinship obligation to accede to her request.
Though force was used, the physician did not use a "destructive pessary" or
knead the woman's uterus. The presumptive fetus was called a seed, not a baby,
or a person.

THE GREEK MEDICAL ETHICS OF ABORTION

Greek medical treatises on fetal development or viability did not describe the
fetus as a person.[43] Nor did Greek physicians describe embryos that they examined as a source of pollution in the sense that other human corpses were
"polluted."[44] Child abandonment, at the discretion of the husband, was practiced to limit family size, select gender, or destroy deformed infants.[45] For these
reasons, it is difficult to read the *Oath's* words on destructive pessaries as a disavowal of abortion as killing of a fetal person, in the current sense of the abortion debate.

The fetal-life argument against abortion would not be written until 200 years
after the *Oath* was written.[46] At about 100 BCE, an inscription on the shrine to
the fertility god Agdistis may have taken wording from the *Oath* and applied it to
all men, notably without specifying physicians: "Let men and women slave and
free, when coming into this shrine swear by all the gods that they will not turn to
nor recommend to others nor have a hand in love-charms, abortives, or contraceptives."[47] The fusing of a fetal-life argument with the idea of a physician's duty
not to destroy a fetal person was not written until the first century CE, a half

millennium after the *Oath* was written. Scribonius Largus, a first century Roman, claimed that the prohibition against abortion was an injunction not to do harm. He argued that killing an embryo, with its unfulfilled promise of becoming a person, was worse than murder.[48] Fifty years later, Soranus argued that medicine's role was to "guard and preserve what has been engendered by nature." He cited "Likewise, I will not give a destructive pessary" as a more restrictive: "I will give no one an abortive." Nevertheless, he said that medical abortion could be justified, "with discrimination, not to a person who wished to destroy the embryo because of adultery or out of consideration for youthful beauty; but to prevent subsequent danger in birth."[49] The full direct text of the *Oath* was by this time lost, and our text dates from 500 CE. From then, it would be another 500 years before the abortion passage was taken up again.

Medieval church scholars brought the *Oath* out of library archives and into public consciousness. As they did so, they rewrote the abortion passage. From the twelfth to the sixteenth century, the abortion passage evolved from a narrow disavowal of pessaries to a more comprehensive pledge including: "Likewise, I will not give a woman an abortifacient," or the even broader "Likewise, I will not give a woman an abortifacient from above or below."[50]

Modern translations continued this restrictive interpretive tradition. One widely used early-twentieth-century translation euphemistically and incorrectly suggested that abortion was illegal in ancient Greece: "I will perform no operation of a criminal purpose, even if solicited; far less suggest it."[51] In 1943, Edelstein's translated this passage to read, "I will not give to a woman an abortive remedy."[52] He argued that a philosophical sect wrote *Oath* and thus laid the foundation for medical ethics to disavow medical abortion. Ironically, Edelstein claimed the *Oath* as an ancient text against medical abortions even as he marginalized the anti–medical abortion ethic by attributing it to a small group of philosophers rather than to the mainstream of medicine.[53] Edelstein's version was discussed by the United State's Supreme Court 1973 *Roe vs. Wade* decision, which rejected it, in part, because it did not represent the views of ancient physicians.[54]

Notwithstanding the many variant translations, all of the passages begin with the word "likewise." This word links the disavowal of an abortive pessary with the preceding disavowal of a deadly drug. Kass asserts that in this way, a physician "refuses to participate directly in ending a life whether in the fullness of days or on the way to birth."[55] His conclusion rests on the premise that the "deadly drug" passage refers to a practice like modern medical euthanasia and that the passage on destructive pessaries refers to a comprehensive disavowal of abortions as killing fetal persons. That conclusion projects modern passions and ideas onto ancient Greece. It seems more likely that "likewise" links two vows proclaiming that physicians will not disrupt the social order either by murder or by undermining the authority of the heads of households.[56]

✳   ✳   ✳

CASE 7.1 Sophi appeared to be about seventeen years old when two refugees carried her into the refugee camp hospital on a makeshift bamboo stretcher. She was Cambodian. At the time, I was medical director of the 50,000-person refugee camp located on the Thai-Cambodian border that she called home. A self-taught midwife had tried to abort a pregnancy by kneading Sophi's uterus. This widely used method of abortion attempts to crush the fetus, break the membranes enclosing it, or separate the placenta from the uterus. Sophi's uterus, which felt like it had contained a four-month fetus, had ruptured. The torn uterus bled freely into her abdomen, and her blood pressure was rapidly falling.

Contraception and abortion are contentious topics in refugee medicine. Many donors forbid funds going to organizations that perform abortions. The relief authorities forbid birth control pills, contraceptive injections, and abortions to women in the refugee camps. Our medical team was given a few hundred condoms every month to prevent disease in a refugee camp of 50,000 persons. Refugees would use the condoms, hang them out to dry, and reuse them until they broke.

A physician from Hippocrates' time would have recognized Sophi. Like most women seeking unskilled abortions, she was young and poor.[57] Like many, she was dispossessed by war. In Medea's voice, Euripides described a woman's view of the life of a refugee in this way:

> May the gods save me from becoming a stateless refugee dragging out an intolerable life in desperate helplessness! That is the most pitiful of all griefs; death is better. Should such a day come to me, I pray for death first. Of all pains and hardships, none is worse than to be deprived of your native land.[58]

An ancient Greek physician would have seen Sophi as a healthy, pregnant woman, but there is no evidence that he would have seen her as carrying a living person. Given that she did not have a guardian and that the physicians of the period believed there were several ways to cause an abortion, it is not clear how he would have answered her request for an abortion. The evidence suggests that her health would have been his first consideration.

Sophi was one among hundreds of millions of women without access to contraception.[59] In the refugee camp, sexual barter for the necessities of life was common; rape was prevalent and went unpunished. Modern relief authorities controlled the kind of medical care Sophi could receive and withheld contraceptives and the means for a safe medical abortion. As with her counterparts in ancient Greece, the local midwife offered an ineffective and unsafe abortion. On that day, Sophi was one of 53,000 women in developing countries who had unsafe abortions, and one of the 200 who would die from that procedure. In her death, she evaded the risk of chronic pelvic pain, infertility, future miscarriage, or pregnancy outside the uterus from lay abortions.

The modern abortion debate is largely between those who maintain that abortion is wrong because it kills a fetal-person and those who hold that the decision to continue or end a pregnancy belongs to the pregnant woman. Neither view was prominent in Greece of 400 BCE. Opponents of medical abortion have altered this passage and elevated it above other passages of the *Oath*. Thus, it has become an icon rather than one passage from a human document of its time that tacitly accepts slavery, limits professional training to men, and invokes Apollo. It is most likely that the moral echoes of the *Oath's* words on "destructive pessaries" speak with those who argue that a woman's husband or parents may rightfully speak on her behalf. This ancient Greek view on the status of women does not add much to resolving the debate about medical abortion in our time.

NOTES

1. See Pellegrino and Thomasma 204. May 92. Veatch RM, "Medical Oaths and Codes: Ethical Analysis," in Reich 1428, 1430. Mall D. "Death and the Rhetoric of Unknowing," in Horan and Mall 650. Carrick says that this passage refers to all abortions but that the actual practice of physicians was diverse (98, 174–6). Ironically, the intensity of the contemporary abortion debate has led to two bioethicists to vary the *Oath* by omitting any abortion passage so that the version will be "widely accepted" (Pellegrino and Thomasma 206).

2. Jonsen says this passage is not clear in its meaning or intent, given uncertainty about who wrote the passage, its restriction to a single abortion technique, and the lack of a commentary elaborating on its meaning ([1998] 285).

3. Verhey A. The doctor's oath—And a Christian swearing it. Linacre Quarterly 1984;51(2):139–58.

4. Value of Life Committee. "The 1995 Restatement of the Oath of Hippocrates, circa 400 BC." National Catholic Bioethics Center, Boston, MA 02135 (available at www.ncbcenter.org.html).

5. *Dislocation of the Womb* (Lefkowitz MR, Fant MB); *Displacement of the Womb* (Lefkowitz MR, Fant MB); *Hysterical Suffocation* (Lefkowitz MR, Fant MB).

6. *Epidemic I; fourteen cases: Case V.*

7. *Diseases of Women I;11* (Hippocrates [1975] 577).

8. Demand finds twenty-seven certain cases of elective abortion and an equal number of possible cases in *Diseases of Women* and *Nature of Women* (Demand 58–9).

9. Hanson AE. "Continuity and Change; Three Case studies in Hippocratic Gynecological Therapy and Theory," in Pomeroy (1991) 73–110.

10. *Epidemics 7:74.*

11. *On the Diseases of Women I:67* in Hanson, op. Cit, in Pomeroy (1991) 80.

12. *The Dangerous First and Sixth 40-Day Periods During Pregnancy; Women's Illnesses.* (Lefkowitz MR, Fant MB.); *Women's Illnesses* (Lefkowitz MR, Fant MB.); *Diseases of Women I;21;25* (Hippocrates [1975] 579).

13. *On the Diseases of Women I:70* in Hanson, op. Cit, in Pomeroy (1991) 93.

14. *On the Diseases of Women 1.72* (Hippocrates [1975] 568).

15. *On the Diseases of Women 1.67* in Blundell 110.

16. The following cases plausibly refer to mortal uterine infections: *Epidemics I; fourteen cases: case xi; Epidemics III; cases x, xi, xii; Epidemics III; (sixteen cases): cases II, XIV; and Epidemics 7:74.* The following aphorisms discuss this matter: "If a pregnant woman have erysipelas of the womb she will die," (*Aphorisms V:43*). "Inflammation of the rectum and of the womb produces stranguary as do suppurative conditions of the kidneys,"(*Aphorisms V:58*). See also *Prorrhetic I:80.* There are also accounts of surviving uterine infection (e.g., *Epidemics 5:13; Diseases of Women I:2*).

17. *On the Nature of Women 32* (Blundell 109). It is not clear whether information about oral abortifacents in the Greek medical works was intended to guide the use of such material or to simply alert physicians to abortion as an effect of these widely used substances or explain how midwives or herb sellers used such agents.

18. Lloyd (1983) 76, and King 178.

19. *Diseases of Women I; Seed; Nature of the Child.* Demand 14–70, 167; Lloyd (1983)62–105. Appendix A dates the gynecological treatises. Substantial material on the treatment of women is found in other treatises as well.

20. *On Superfetation;*32–3 (Blundell 105); *Diseases of Women I:11* (Hippocrates [1975] 577); *Epidemics* 2:6:29.

21. *Epidemics I: (fourteen cases); case 4 and 5.*

22. Blundell 111.

23. *Places in man 47; Dislocation of the Womb* (Lefkowitz MR, Fant MB.).

24. *Women's Illnesses; Hysterical Suffocation; Displacement of the Womb* (Lefkowitz MR, Fant MB.).

25. *Displacement of the Womb* (Lefkowitz MR, Fant MB.).

26. *Epidemics* 7:6.

27. Carrick 119 citing Littré. Oeuvres vol 8:171.

28. Demand 68–70, 132–33.

29. Pomeroy (1975) 72–84; (1998) 93–8; Blundell 135–45.

30. Euripides. *Hippolytus* 293–6.

31. King 172–82; Lloyd (1983) 73–4. As assistants during surgery on women, women appeared to have jobs that were analogous to those of men who were surgical assistants or apprenticed physicians (Jouanna 89–91). Within families, women performed basic nursing care under the direction of midwives, nurses, or physicians. Female nurses administered remedies as independent healers and in collaboration with physicians (King 158–71). It is possible that the Greek medical treatises' descriptions of dietetic and herbal therapies were written compilations of the oral lore of women healers. Langholf 108.

32. *Hysterical Suffocation* (Lefkowitz, Fant MB.).

33. Lloyd [1983] 70–2. *Womens Illnesses* (Lefkowitz MR, Fant MB.).

34. Blundell 114; King 16, 22, 181; Pomeroy 62–5. Generally, older widows who had an independent trade or stigmatized women lacked guardians and were known by their own names (King 60; Pomeroy [1975] 72–74.)

35. Demand 6, 12, 41, 45, 61–2.

36. Cohen 133–70.

37. Sophocles. *Oedipus the King* (1984) 1645–50.

38. For example, in *Epidemics I and III*—the oldest *Epidemics*—the men are Hermocrates, Philistes, Cleanactides, Meton, Crito, Philiscus, Silenus, and Herophon. The women are the nameless wife of Philinus, the wife of Hicetas, the wife of Epicrates, the wife of Dromeades, a woman who was one of the house [probably a slave] of Pantimedes, and the maiden daughter of Euryanax.

39. Pomeroy (1975) 33.

40. *Generation 6* (Hippocrates [1950]).

41. Aeschylus. *The Eumenides* 665–71.

42. *On the Nature of the Child* 13.

43. *Eight-Months Child* 12; *On the Nature of the Child* 14, 16–22; *Fleshes* 19 (two places); *Epidemics* 2;6:iv and above case note on an abortion.

44. von Staden H. The discovery of the body: Human dissection and its cultural contexts in ancient Greece. Yale J Biol and Med 1992;223–41. *Fleshes* 19.

45. Edwards ML. The cultural context of deformity in the ancient Greek world: "Let there be a law that no deformed child shall be reared." Ancient Hist Bull 1996;10(3–4):79–92. Amundsen DW. "Medicine and the Birth of Defective Children: Approaches of the Ancient World," in McMillan, Engelhardt, and Spicker S. 3–32.

46. Carrick 115–46; Kudlien F. Medical ethics and popular ethics in Greece and Rome. Clio Med 1970;5:91–121.

47. The inscription goes on to say, "A man is not to have relationships with the wife of another whether a free woman or a married slave, or with a boy, or with a virgin or to counsel this to another." This wording is evocative of the *Oath* but also reflects a more ascetic strain of thought that postdates it. Campbell ML. The Oath: An investigation of the injunction prohibiting physician–patient sexual relations. Perspect Biol Med 1989;32:300–8.

48. Pellegrino Ed, Pellegrino AA. Humanism and ethics in Roman medicine: Translation and commentary on a text of Scribonius Largus. Lit Med 1988;7:22–38. Hamilton JS. Scribonius Largus on the medical profession. Bull Hist Med 1986;60:209–16.

49. Temkin O. "The Idea of Respect for Life in the History of Medicine," in Temkin, Frankena, and Kadish 3. Translation slightly reworded for readability.

50. Jones (1924) 23–25. Tutten T. Receptions of the Hippocratic Oath in the Renaissance: The prohibition of abortion as a case study in reception. J Hist Med Allied Sci, 1996;51:456–83.

51. Smith DC. The Hippocratic Oath and Modern Medicine. J Hist Med Allied Sci, 1996;51:494.

52. Edelstein L. The Hippocratic Oath: Text, Translation, and Interpretation," in (Temkin and Temkin 3–64). As far as I can determine, the Pythagorean anti-abortion position seems to have been articulated by neo-Pythagoreans centuries after the *Oath* was written. There is a long gap in the literature between Pythagoreans ca. 500 BC and the anti-abortion position articulated by neo-Pythagoreans centuries after the *Oath* was written.

53. The problems with Edelstein's view are discussed in Chapter 3. It is noteworthy that Justice Blackmum in *Roe vs Wade* precisely referred to this aspect of Edelstein's position. Citing Edelstein, Blackmun wrote that the *Oath*'s injunction against abortion represented the position of "only a small segment of Greek opinion and that it certainly was not accepted by all ancient physicians" (Roe *vid supra* at 131).

54. *Roe vs. Wade*, 410 U. S. 113 (1973).

55. Kass 234.

56. It is interesting to consider why the abortion passage follows, rather than precedes, the passage on deadly drugs. Contemporary bioethicists tend to proceed from the beginning of life to the end of life. The *Oath* proceeds from the social world to the private world. Murder is a crime against society. Abortion would transgress against the male head of the house. In this reading (and assuming the reading of the surgery passage is correct), the abortion passage is properly located at the threshold of the house before the purification on entering the house. This would be where the head of the house would invite the physician to enter, and it would be an appropriate place for the physician to promise to not transgress against the privileges of the head of the household.

57. Mundigo and Indriso.

58. Euripides (Vellacott translation), *Medea 642–51*.

59. World Health Organization. World Health Day/Safe Motherhood, 7 April 1998: Address Unsafe Abortion. who.int/archives/whday/en/pages1998/whd98_10.html and safemotherhood.org/facts_and_figures/unsafe_abortion_fact.html.

8

INTEGRITY

IN A PURE AND HOLY WAY, I WILL GUARD MY LIFE AND MY
TECHNÉ[1] [ART AND SCIENCE.]

Modern readers tend to hear this passage as proposing a morally aloof, insular, even priestly medical professionalism. Yet ancient Greek physicians were practical workers in a society that expected them to be engaged citizens rather than ascetics who stood apart. Von Staden's authoritative analysis of this passage examines and successfully resolves the apparent paradox between the apparently inward-looking sense of these words and a life of professional engagement with society.[2] It is helpful to read this passage one half at a time.

IN A PURE AND HOLY WAY . . .

The word *holy* had a different meaning in ancient Greece than it does today.[3] Today, it refers to "the radical otherness of God's inner world . . . and designates certain places, times, objects and priestly persons as set apart and sacrosanct, in some sense charged with God's own holy presence."[4] Our culture tends to view the everyday world as fundamentally separated from a holy dominion.

By contrast, ancient Greece was a sacralized culture in which the natural world was suffused with the holy. Activities of daily life, and not simply worship, took place in a world that was at once holy and natural.[5] A daily life lived in a holy way promoted justice (*diké*) so that the natural and social worlds would flourish.[6] Unholy acts undermined the natural and social worlds. Holy activities, thoughts, or words were part of everyday activities rather than being reserved for special times, rituals, or activities. They were distinguished from those that were "sacred" (i.e., forbidden to all but priests) and those that were "profane" (forbidden to all). A person engaged in healing, midwifery, or soldiering was "holy" if he or she performed those activities in a manner that was consonant with the moral traditions for that work. For example, though soldiers were allowed to kill and enslave defeated civilians during war, it was profane for Ajax to enter Athena's temple to enslave the princess Cassandra who had taken sanctuary there after her city was defeated.[7] Because of this transgression, the victorious army was destroyed. In this sense of a "holy life," the *Oath* does not set a physician apart; rather, it proclaims and defines the necessity of a morally engaged professional life.

In a similar way, the vow to be "pure" describes how the physician will engage the world rather expressing a pledge of ascetic distance from society. The concept of "pure" was central to Greek society and medicine; it referred to a state of being free from moral pollution.[8] Acting or thinking profanely could pollute a person. A person could acquire pollution by touch. For example, touching a corpse or a murderer caused one to become polluted. Temkin remarks that Greeks saw the transmission of pollution as an explanation for contagion.[9] If so, purification had both a medical and a moral significance. Being polluted was an offense against the moral order, the natural world, and human society. Rituals of purification such as bathing, being anointed, prayer, or offering sacrifices could remove pollution. Once purified, a person could ask to enter a temple or have prayers heard. The physician's vow to keep "in a pure way" is a pledge to strive to remain free of pollution. Purity and a holy life were thus intertwined, not in an ascetically disengaged life, but rather though a well-lived life.

Von Staden cites an inscription on an Asclepian temple from 300 BCE as illustrating the relationship between *pure* and *holy* for healers, "Pure must the person be who goes inside the fragrant temple. And purity is to think holy thoughts."[10] It may be objected that Von Staden is overreaching in that the inscription may have been directed to sick persons; to wit, that an illness could be cured only when the person was purified and living in a holy way. Socrates noted, however, that the "purifications which doctors and diviners use, and their fumigations with drugs magical or medicinal, as well as their washings and lustral sprinklings, have all one and the same object, which is to make a man pure both in body and soul."[11] In this view, physicians, like patients, would have to be pure in order to employ the tools of healing. It seems plausible that Hippocratic healers, like temple healers, would have had some words or rituals of purification as they entered patients' houses. Perhaps this passage from the *Oath* was part of that ritual.

Holiness and purity are not synonymous with virtues. Virtues were attributes of character that led individuals to lead a good life or to rectify injustice.[12] Greeks admired many personal virtues, including courage, moderation in appetites, decorum, friendliness, mild temper, and prudence. There were also social virtues: greatness of soul, generosity of spirit, hospitality, and a sense of justice. Pellegrino offers a list of virtues for the modern physician: fidelity to trust, keeping promises, benevolence, effacement of self-interest, compassion and caring, intellectual honesty, justice in the sense of treating one's patients equally according to their special needs, and prudence, defined as having a deliberative and discerning judgment.[13] "Holy" referred to living in an upright manner. "Virtues" were dispositions by which each person could live in an upright manner that helped a society to flourish in accord with the underlying moral order.[14] "Purification" was a means by which past transgressions could be left behind. Together, the three concepts informed, enabled, and rectified moral living.

. . . I WILL GUARD MY LIFE, MY ART, AND MY SCIENCE

The vow to "guard my life, my art, and my science" acknowledges that one must be self-reflective to live a moral personal and professional life as a physician. The *Oath* does not presume that a physician has moral integrity. Vigilance guaranteed by an oath is required. The threats a physician must guard against are not specified but presumably include temptations or coercion to act in ways that do not benefit the ill, or that allow injustice, harm medical education, or breach promises to one's teachers.[15] The fact that the *Oath* requires a physician to swear to be vigilant to guard his own integrity highlights the fact that a physician who is not morally vigilant risks practicing medicine in a way that is not holy.

The physician's moral vigilance must look to "my life and *techné* [art and science]." By these words the *Oath* emphasized that the physician's personal and professional (*techné*) lives must be morally coherent, though it does not assert that the same moral obligations apply to each of them.[16] The *Oath's* closing also refers to the moral unity of the personal and professional life, "may it be granted to me to enjoy the benefits both of life and of *techné*" [art and science]. (see Chapter 13). In that later passage, the *Oath* builds from this passage asserting the moral importance of their unity to add the Greek belief that a good life is the most secure foundation for a happy life. Perhaps more important for professional ethics, a good life is one that achieves excellence in its purpose, an excellence that must include the exercise of virtues that are instrumental to one's life work.[17] Thus, in its separate uses of "life and *techné*," the *Oath* commits the physician's entire moral life to that which is required to be a good physician.

This comprehensive vow is intensely personalized in its unique three-fold use of the first person: "In a pure and holy way, *I* will guard *my* life and *my* techné [art and science]." As von Staden notes, the triple proclaiming of the first person, to an even greater degree than the other elements of the *Oath*, seems to suggest that this passage was a self-transforming ritual of purification itself.[18] The placement of this passage at the very threshold to the patient's house emphasizes the ideal of medicine as a moral profession.

✳ ✳ ✳

CASE 8.1 Isaac is an older friend, a dignified, well-read gentleman. One day he said to me, "I want your advice on how to write a letter to my doctor. She prescribed a medicine for osteoarthritis in my hips. Soon after starting it, my legs began to swell. I told my doctor about this, and she gave me some pills to re-move the excess fluid. The drug damaged my kidneys and now I may need to go on an artificial kidney machine. She should have known that a person of my age could get kidney failure from that drug. I trusted her judgment that this medica-tion was right for me. I feel that she let me down."

This chapter has focused on what the *Oath* said about the importance of a physician's integrity to medical work. Professional integrity is crucial both to fostering a trusting physician–patient relationship as well as to maintaining trust between society and the institutions and activities of medicine. Does this pas-sage from the *Oath* still speak to the medical ethics of integrity? There are sev-eral ways to consider how this passage might address the issues in Isaac's treatment.

One could focus, as Isaac does, on the integrity of his physician. She had prescribed a non-steroidal anti-inflammatory drug (NSAID). Such drugs are often recommended for treating arthritis pain. Isaac felt that his physician had erred either in selecting the medication or in failing to monitor him for a known and serious side effect. Isaac correctly believes that a physician who is negligent in keeping informed about how to optimally use the tools of medicine to benefit and not harm a patient lacks a kind of integrity with regard to the physician's pledge to "benefit of the ill." There is no evidence, especially given the widespread use of these drugs for people like Isaac, to suggest that this physician's prescription of this drug was inattentive. If Isaac's physician's failed to detect his problem because she was seeing too many patients, this might indicate a lack of integrity in which Isaac's health was endangered by the physician's (or clinic's) desire for high revenues.[19] Not every error or bad outcome necessarily signifies that a lack of professional integrity, however. (see Chapter 9).

The physicians who worked at the behest of pharmaceutical companies to develop these drugs also shaped the clinical decision that resulted in this drug's being prescribed to Isaac. To understand how their integrity might be related to Isaac's injury requires some history. Physicians and drug companies have long known that older people like Isaac need better arthritis medications, and in the 1960s, NSAIDs seemed a promising development. They neither had the addictive potential of narcotics nor caused bone degeneration like the corticosteroids. However, long before these drugs came to market, physician-scientists knew that NSAIDs caused kidney disease.[20] Researchers soon discovered that older people were especially at risk of serious kidney disease. In 1974, the New England Journal warned that a new NSAID was "best not used" in the elderly.[21] By 1982, 70 million prescriptions for NSAIDs were filled in the United States, and more than half of these were for the twelve percent of people over 65 years old.[22] By 1984, independent researchers were urging "extreme caution" in using NSAIDs in high-risk groups, including people with common diseases of the elderly.[23]

Though these drugs were being marketed, sold, and prescribed to elderly persons, only two percent of the subjects in NSAID arthritis studies conducted between 1987 and 1990 were elderly. Corporate-sponsored researchers often failed to support their claims of the superior safety.[24] By 1990, NSAIDs accounted for twenty-five percent of all drug side effects.[25] The issue of integrity is raised by medical research that heralds benefits by studies designed to avoid assessing the serious risks to those who will probably use that drug and to whom that drug is marketed. Unfortunately, this problem with professional integrity is common in corporate-sponsored pharmaceutical research.

Drug companies provide more funding for medical research in the United States than the federal government.[26] Some of this money is spent in corporate labs; some goes to university medical researchers. Some university researchers also receive speaking fees, consultancies, equipment, stocks, or stock options that fluctuate in value according to a company's profits. These forms of compensation can vary in worth from a few hundred dollars to more than a hundred thousand dollars per year.[27] Three-fourths of the professors who accept such material consideration say that it is important to their work. Drug companies even hire advertising agencies to conduct pharmaceutical research.[28] In short, researchers conduct a great deal of research while having significant financial stakes in the outcome of the research or in maintaining an ongoing pecuniary relationship with a pharmaceutical manufacturer. Such ties are morally problematic if they adversely affect the conduct of research or harm patients. Unfortunately, they do.

Corporate drug development has two aims: to make a profit and to promote health. These valid interests can conflict with each other, and such strains can extend to the conduct and reporting of biomedical research. Corporate-sponsored research tends to exaggerate the benefits of a specific drug, minimize its harms, understate costs, and promote the use of a newer treatment over a comparably effective and less expensive therapy.[29] Biases are designed into the studies. In NSAID research, for example, the studies were done on younger persons who were at lower risk of side effects than those who would be the major users of the drugs. A new drug may be compared with an unfairly low dose of a competing drug. A drug may shine against a placebo when it is no better than an inexpensive conventional treatment. Test scores or lab values can create the appearance of benefit when a person's health is not changed. The data from this distorted research are then disseminated to shape clinical decisions, such as the decision to use the NSAID for Isaac. Physicians who accept remuneration from corporations are much more likely to defend a controversial drug than those who do not accept this kind of support.[30]

Corporate sponsors favorably "spin" and disseminate research findings. Corporate writers often write scientific papers that respected research physicians review and then sign as the authors. Corporations have threatened to sever relationships with researchers who do not deliver favorable findings, and occasionally to sue researchers or medical journals if unfavorable, albeit accurate, data are published.[31] Data files of corporate clinical studies are often closed, thereby preventing independent assessments of their findings. The research findings form a curriculum for professional education, including Doughnut Rounds. (see Chapter 4.)

Is it fair, however, to argue that this passage from the *Oath* can speak to the issue of the integrity of modern corporate-sponsored research? It would be hard to argue that ancient Greeks could have anticipated modern corporate drug research. Even so, do the *Oath's* words on integrity apply to the creation and dissemination of medical knowledge in ancient Greece? If so, they can speak to us today. As noted in Chapter 4, the ancient Greek idea of experiments did not involve clinical trials with multiple subjects. Instead, each patient was given the best therapy possible, and by these individual cases, the physician tried to discern how to improve the practice. The ancient treatises stress the physician's duty to accurately and fairly note observations upon which inferences and subsequent treatment recommendations were made. As the author of *On Ancient Medicine* wrote, "if anyone were able to light upon the truth by experiment . . . he would always be able to make the best pronouncements of all."[32] The entire corpus of the practical casework of ancient Greek medicine is essentially the records of these experiments.

Modern physicians use different research methodologies but have essentially the same goal: to accurately collect and describe their experiments. They go to great lengths to acquire accurate data by randomly assigning research subjects to receive one drug or the other and not informing researchers which person has received which therapy until after the clinical outcomes have been collected. Falsely reporting procedures for randomizing patients, the treatments that were given, how the researchers were blinded, or the measurements of results are all acts that are censured as research fraud. Ironically, though numerous studies show that corporate sponsorship distorts the design and dissemination of research, reforms for this problem are largely stalled.[33] Furthermore, even if regulatory reforms were implemented, compliance with the spirit of those reforms would squarely engage the integrity of physician-researchers. As Isaac's case shows, the integrity of the design of research and of the way that research findings are disseminated directly affects the patient's well-being.

NOTES

1. Von Staden leaves "*techné*" in Greek. I have rendered it as "art and science." Chadwick renders *techné* as "art" (Hippocrates [1950]). Jones translates it as "Science" (Hippocrates [1923]). *Techné* refers to the purposeful and discerning application of the natural science of medicine. As a science, it includes universality, generalizability, teachability, precision, and concern with explanation (Nussbaum 95–121). As an art, it includes wisdom and insight. *Techné* is more than the unreflective practice of an acquired skill or tradition. It is unlike *tuché*, the luck or coincidence that lies behind a testimonial on behalf of the worth of a charlatan.

2. von Staden H. "In a Pure and Holy Way": Personal and professional conduct in the Hippocratic Oath. J Hist Med Allied Sci 1996;51:404–37.

3. There were medical cults, such as the group that probably wrote the medical treatise entitled *Law*, that use *holy* in a cultic sense: "Things that are holy are revealed only to men who are holy. The profane may not learn them until they have been initiated into the mysteries of science. (*Law V*)" See (Hippocrates 1923) note by Jones 273, 5. There is no evidence that this was a dominant view of Hippocratic-era physicians.

4. Childress and MacQuarrie 269.

5. Eliade 110, 116.

6. Pearson 90–160.

7. Euripides. *The Trojan Women* 68–85.

8. Adkins 86–102. Parker extensively discusses this.

9. Temkin O. "An Historical Analysis of the Concept of Infection," in Boas et al., 123–47 at 125. Unfortunately Temkin did not develop the grounds for this remark.

10. Von Staden, op. cit.

11. Plato. *Cratylus 405a-b.*

12. I accept von Staden, who reads this as a pledge to act in an honorable way, though others read it as a promise to maintain a virtuous character (Pellegrino and Thomasma 120). Pellegrino is careful, though, to not reduce the *Oath* simply to a pledge to have virtue; he emphasizes that the *Oath* as a whole includes responsibilities and rules as well (Pellegrino 107, 115–6, 126–9).

13. Pellegrino 125–6. The concept of prudence is elaborated on in Pellegrino 130–49.

14. Nussbaum MC. Non-relative virtues: An Aristotelian approach. Midwest Studies in Philosophy 1998;13:32–53.

15. von Staden H. "Character and Competence I: Personal and Professional Conduct in Greek Medicine," in Flashar and Jouanna 157–210.

16. Pellegrino 107.

17. MacIntyre 146–164,204–226 esp. 219–21.

18. The personally transforming nature of the swearing the *Oath* is discussed more extensively in the Afterword.

19. Rodwin.

20. Stewart JH.

21. Mills JA. Nonsteroidal anti-inflammatory drugs. N Engl J Med 1974;290: 780–4.

22. Rochon PA, Fortin PR, Dear KBG, et al. Reporting of age data in clinical trials of arthritis: Deficiencies and solutions. Arch Intern Med 1993;153:243–8.

23. Clive DM, Stolf JS. Renal syndromes associated with nonsteroidal anti-inflammatory drugs. N Engl J Med 1984;310:563–72.

24. Rochon PA, Fortin PR, Dear KBG, et al. *vid supra.*

25. Rochon PA, Gurwitz JH, Simms RW et al. A study of manufacturer-supported trials of nonsteroidal anti-inflammatory drugs in the treatment of arthritis. Arch Intern Med 1994;154:157–63.

26. Rettig RA. The industrialization of clinical research. Health Aff 2000;19: 129–46.

27. Boyd EA, Bero LA. Assessing faculty financial relationships with industry: A case study. JAMA 2000;284:2209–14. Campbell EG, Seashore L, Blumenthal D. Looking a gift horse in the mouth: Corporate gifts supporting life sciences research. JAMA 1998;279:995–9.

28. Peterson M. Madison Avenue. Plays Growing Role in the Business of Drug Research. *New York Times,* 2002;(November 22): A1, C4.

29. Stelfox HT, Chua G, O'Rourke K, Detsky AS. Conflict of interest in the debate over calcium-channel antagonists. N Engl J Med 1998;338:101–6.

30. Bodenheimer T. Uneasy alliance: Clinical investigators and the pharmaceutical industry. New Engl J Med 2000;342:1539–44. Friedberg M, Saffran B, Stinson TJ, et al. Evaluation of conflict of interest in economic analyses of new drugs' use in oncology. JAMA 1999;282:1453–7. Rero LA, Rennie D. Influences on the quality of published drug studies. Int J Technol Assess Health Care 1996;12:209–37. Kjaergard LL, Bodil AN. Association between competing interests and authors' conclusions: Epidemiological study of randomized clinical trials published in the BMJ. BMJ 2002;325:249–53.

31. Nathan DG, Weatherall DJ. Academic freedom in clinical research. N Engl J Med 2002;347:1368–70.

32. *Tradition in Medicine 20,24.* Translation from Hippocrates 1950. Loeb title of same treatise is *On Ancient Medicine.*

33. Schulman KA, Seils DM, Timbie JW, et al. A national survey of provisions in clinical trial agreements between medical schools and industry sponsors. N Engl J Med 2002;347:1335–41. Some medical journals now require that researchers show that they are independent of corporate control before a paper will be accepted for publication. (Davidoff F, De Angelis CD, Drazen JM, et al. Sponsorship, authorship, and accountability. Ann Intern Med 2001;135:463–5.) Some propose that companies give funds for researching a particular drug to an independent group that would choose a research design and researchers to evaluate the drug.

9

ERRORS

I WILL NOT CUT, AND CERTAINLY NOT THOSE SUFFERING
FROM STONE, BUT I WILL CEDE THIS TO MEN WHO ARE
PRACTITIONERS OF THIS ACTIVITY.

This passage is puzzling. It reads like a vow to forswear surgery by physicians who proudly and aggressively performed many kinds of surgical procedures (see Table 9–1). Numerous Greek medical texts discussed indications for surgery and described surgical techniques (including how to vary the incising stroke to minimize pain during different kinds of operations), cutting instruments (cold or cauterizing, ostentatious or simply workmanlike), how to illuminate surgical incisions, market surgical skills, and use surgical assistants.[1] Authors recommended surgical instruction early in one's medical education and suggested military service as the best place to learn trauma surgery.[2] Greek physicians left an enduring impact on surgery.

Twenty-three centuries after the Greek surgical works were written, the nineteenth-century French surgeon Jules Le Coeur of Caen wrote, "We must return to the practice of the Ancients," as he recommended using sterilizing agents on compound fractures.[3] Greek advice about how long to wait before attempting to drain purulent fluid from around a lung was debated throughout the nineteenth century and ultimately vindicated during the influenza epidemic of the early twentieth century.[4] Ironically, many of the Greek sur-

TABLE 9.1 Ancient Greek Surgery

Trephining (cutting down to, or through bones):

- Skull bones to allow drainage to prevent abscesses or to drain pus or blood[49]
- Bone abscesses by directly incising into a bone or removing bone[50]
- Exploratory debridement to assess for skull fractures[51]

Surgery for trauma and to remove spears, knives, etc.[52]
Amputation[53]
Excising exposed bone in open fractures[54]
Draining empyema (pus collected inside the chest cavity, outside the lung)[55]
Incising traumatic abscesses of the abdominal wall[56]
Incising rectal abscesses and excising or ligating hemorrhoids[57]
Incising into the kidney to drain abscesses and stones[58]
Hooking bladder stones with urethral catheters[59]
Removing fluid:

- Draining pleural effusions[60]
- Abdominal paracentesis[61]
- Arthrocentesis of the knee[62]
- Multiple incisions for edema[63]

Removing a retained, dead fetus[64]
Removing polyps of the nose and pharynx[65]
Tooth extractions[66]

---

gical procedures listed on Table 9.1 seem to be proscribed by the *Oath* and yet remain part of medical practice today.[5] So, what does "I will not cut . . ." mean, either as a characterization of ancient medicine or as an ethical statement within the *Oath*?

CONTENDING INTERPRETATIONS

The great Hippocratic scholar Emile Littré was the first academician to tackle the meaning of this passage. He translated it as, "I will not practice surgery for stone; I will leave this to people who do that." His translation restricts the scope of the passage to "surgery for stone" rather than reading it as a general disavowal of surgery, especially surgery for stones. Though linguists do not accept the restrictive translation, many commentators tacitly accept it and narrowly debate the kind of stones that are being referred to. Veatch asserts it was gallstones.[6] Wangensteen said they were kidney stones, though *Internal Affections* describes cutting into the kidney to flush stones out. That treatise described "violent pain" while passing "sand through the urethra" and commended putting a hot pack over the kidney and "when the affected area swells up and becomes raised, incise immediately over the kidney, draw out the pus, and attend to the sand with diuretics" to induce urination.[7] Murphy also believes *Oath* was referring to kidney stones, though he believes that *Internal Affections* was discussing draining a perinephric abscess.[8] Littré proposes that "stone" referred to "testicle"; "I confess that in this context, I am led to conclude that the reference to 'stone' refers to castration. At least, the taboo on performing such mutilation can be understood without difficulty."[9] He reviews the literature on castration in ancient Greece and suggests that "I will not cut and certainly not those suffering from stone" is a somewhat euphemistic statement of a serious moral obligation to not mutilate in this manner.

In support of Littré's conclusion, the Greek medical writings seem surprisingly reticent about surgery on male genitalia, given that trauma, abscesses, torsion, or tumors of male genitalia are relatively common today and there is no reason that those conditions should have been less common in ancient Greece. Surgery on the male genitalia was within the scope of the technical skills of Greek surgeons, logical given their approaches to similar pathologies on other organs, and would have benefited some men or boys.[10] Perhaps the reticence of the ancient treatises reflects a form of self-censoring on the subject of cutting on male genitalia, or perhaps the texts discussing such surgery were lost or censored later. Unfortunately, the very gravity of the moral claim that castration is taboo raises a new problem with Littré's solution. If this passage referred to a castration taboo, why did it promote referrals to other practitioners?

In the mid–twentieth century, Edelstein made the second notable attempt to reconcile this passage with the surgical proclivity of the Greek physicians. He read the disavowal of surgery as supporting evidence for his belief that a sect of medical philosophers who rejected the pro-surgery position of the medical community of the time wrote the *Oath*.[11] The absence of evidence for the existence of such a group at the time the *Oath* was written neither proves nor disproves this hypothesis. If Edelstein is correct, one could accept that the *Oath's* referral to surgeons was a moral act somewhat akin to the way an avowedly celibate priest might refer a married couple to a marriage counselor.[12] But this pluralistic accommodation with surgery begs the question of what the "stone" language means. If these philosophers disavowed cutting altogether, the disavowal of cutting for stones adds nothing. Or, as with Littré's conclusion, if cutting for stone was especially taboo, why endorse referrals? The logical problems called for a fresh approach.

Kass offered a solution that seems to avoid the paradoxes of Littré's and Edelstein's solutions. He suggests that this vow refers to forswearing to undertake a medical act that is beyond one's competence.[13] Murphy suggests that this moral obligation is especially profound when it comes to highly invasive or dangerous surgery near the kidney.[14] Unfortunately, Kass seems unaware of the robust and risky surgical practice of Greek physicians.[15] He is, however, correct in assuming that not all physicians were equally qualified to perform all procedures. The ancient physicians proclaimed their specialized skills and criticized those who did procedures they were not prepared for. For example, physicians with military experience touted the value of that experience in learning how to perform surgery for trauma and foreign bodies.[16] Nonetheless, there are problems in reading this passage as a vow to stick to one's own areas of competence. Why did it narrowly refer to "cutting" to make the general point that physicians should not practice beyond their sphere of skill when Greek physicians employed many dangerous treatments, including cauterizing wounds or cancers with hot irons, debriding skull fractures, and administering toxic plants? This problem with the Kass conclusion seems less severe than the paradoxes plaguing Littré's and Edelstein's hypotheses.

Littré and Edelstein both use the historical chronology of surgery in their attempts to decode this passage. Edelstein uses the contradiction between the *Oath's* disavowal of surgery and the acceptance of surgery at the time the *Oath* was written to make the case that philosophers wrote the *Oath*. Littré looks to the culture of ancient Greece for support for the view that this passage refers to castration. The history of surgery can be used in a different way to date this passage. The passage gives three hints about its historical setting. First, it does not condemn surgery (as Edelstein implies); on the contrary, referrals are recommended. Second, it seems to regard surgeons as being in a separate kind of practice from the physician who swore this oath. Third, surgery for stone was seen as a special kind of operation. There was a time when these three criteria coincided; however, that time is a couple of centuries after 400 BCE when the *Oath* is supposed to have been written. Assuming that the *Oath* is properly dated, is it possible that this one passage was inserted into the *Oath* during the Roman or early Christian era? A plausible, if circumstantial, case can be made for this hypothesis.

To begin with, "I will not cut" is not representative of Greek thinking in 400 BCE. The medical writings of that time show an undefensive pride in surgery.[17] Non-physician writers of that time, including Plato and Sophocles,[18] accept surgery as a part of a physician's work, even though some persons were recognized as experts in particular procedures. The extensive writings about surgical prowess are entirely unlike the reticence about taboo acts (e.g., giving poison, administering abortive pessaries, or having sexual relations with patients). Although those writings discuss controversies about the relative merits of medical versus surgical approaches to specific conditions,[19] the merits of surgery as a medical skill do not appear to be controversial except in this one passage. "I will not cut" was not a part of Greek medical ethics in 400 BCE.

Second, surgery became a separate specialty during Roman times, several centuries after the *Oath* was written. Though ancient Greek writings show that individual physicians were recognized as especially being especially adept at surgery[20] or certain kinds of surgery, scalpels and hot cutting irons were used by many physicians. The surgery books addressed general practitioners for whom surgery was part of their daily work. The societal definition of surgery as a separate profession, in some cases with legally protected surgical privileges, came later. Withington and Jones each cite Galen (150 CE) as asserting that surgery was a specialized form of medical practice in Rome.[21] Aulus Cornelius Celsus (30 CE) described three specialties: those who prescribe a healthy regimen of diet, exercise, and lifestyle; those who prescribe medicines; and those who practice surgery. He wrote that:

> I have already stated, and all the world knows, there is a third department of medicine, or that which is surgical. Now this, although not excluding medicine and diet, nevertheless employs the hand as its chief curative agent and is, of the three divisions of the healing arts, the one whose beneficial effects are most evident.[22]

Though a physician's disavowal of surgery did not make sense in the *Oath's* time, the preceding quote's respectful account of the specialization of physicians comports with the *Oath's* commendation of referrals, ("I will not cut . . . but I will cede this to men who are practitioners of this activity"). This collegiality resolves the logical contradictions of Edelstein's and Littré's hypotheses.

The acknowledgment of surgical specialists also establishes a foundation for resolving the special caution with regard to surgery on persons who are suffering from stone.

A revolution in surgery for bladder stones occurred about one hundred and fifty years after the *Oath* was written. Celsus credits Ammonius (b. 276 BCE) of Alexandria with inventing difficult and dangerous surgery for directly cutting into the bladder from the front of the lower abdomen and then splitting the stone and removing it from the bladder. This procedure was devised in about 240 BCE, and records suggest that it became widely practiced.[23] The Greek works of the *Oath's* time describe a simpler, less invasive, and less effective procedure of inserting a device through the urethra into the bladder to either snag a stone or press it downward against the perineum to try to remove it with a local incision. The new procedure amply justified a cautious referral to experienced hands within the surgical community. Thus, "I will not cut, and certainly not those suffering from stone, but I will cede this to men who are practitioners of this activity" would be a prudent and understandable statement at a time when surgeons were largely separated from other physicians, after the invention of the new technique for bladder lithotomy.

The first century BCE would be a reasonable estimate of when this passage from the *Oath* would reflect the medical ethic of the time (see Figure 9–1). At that time, the logical contradiction in Edelstein's idea that a physician would both disavow and refer for surgery is not present. Also, in that cutting for stone was not morally taboo like Littré's castration but simply technically difficult and risky, the *Oath's* cautionary commendation for referral for bladder lithotomy is prudent rather than bizarre. Finally, this proposal comports with Kass' speculation that this passage is about ethically using professional referrals to minimize risks to patients. Though logically appealing, this solution now creates a gap of two or three centuries between the alleged writing of the *Oath*[24] and the time when this passage was written.

How might this chronological discrepancy be explained? The ancient Greek medical treatises were translated, mistranslated, copied, and revised for nearly a millennium in a process that inserted and deleted material from many treatises.[25] Only iconic respect would justify believing that the *Oath* was immune to such emending. Furthermore, the Oxyrhynchus papyrus is the oldest extant text of the *Oath*. This papyrus dates to 300 CE, 700 years after *Oath* was written, 500 years after the introduction for the new form of

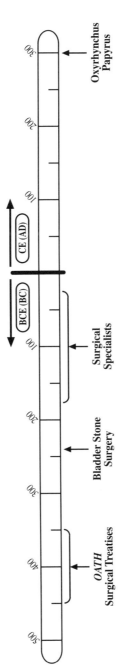

FIGURE 9.1 Key dates in ancient surgery and the *Oath*.

bladder stone surgery, and about 400 years after surgeons separated from their nonsurgical colleagues.[26] If "I will not cut . . . " was inserted into the *Oath* after the invention of bladder lithotomy and the separation of surgeons and before the Oxyrhynchus papyrus, it would appear in all the versions of the text that we know, and time would have allowed the fact of the insertion to be forgotten. We do not have quotations that refer to a surgical passage dating from 400 BCE; in fact, there are no documents prior to about the birth of Jesus referring to any portion of the *Oath*.[27] Though an insertion may be forgotten, there may still be evidence that it occurred, however.

The grammar and composition of the *Oath* may contain additional evidence to clarify this matter. Jones noted a grammatical anachronism in the "cut for stone" passage that distinguished its Greek from that of the rest of the *Oath*. Of this anomaly he said, "It is possible that the degradation of surgery did not take place until Christian times and [this] sentence of *Oath* may well be very late indeed."[28] The surgical passage also disrupts the structure of the *Oath*. It is separate from the other two groups of taboos: abortion and poison, or sexual abuse and keeping secrets.[29] Furthermore, if it is removed, the public ethics stanza and the entry to the clinical encounter are only separated by the ritual of purification of the physician who is at the threshold of entering the patient's house to heal. The *Oath* would then have this appealing and logical flow:

> In a pure and holy way, I will guard my life, my art, and my science.
> Into the households I enter, I will go to benefit the ill.

The possibility that the *Oath* was emended does not diminish it or means that it arrived to us as damaged goods.

Valued things are used, repaired, updated, and restored. The countless variations of the *Oath* of our time bear witness to this regard for the *Oath*. If an older text of the *Oath* were amended by inserting the surgical vow, this would be evidence that the *Oath* was valued and used in 200 BCE. This version would have been used by physicians who practiced some form of nonsurgical "internal medicine" or "hygiene" but who referred patients to their surgical colleagues. A group of such physicians may have simply amended the older *Oath* to adjust for the scope of their practice in their time.[30] If the *Oath* was amended, this change played some role in creating the version that was transmitted to our time, and for that, we should be grateful.

ERROR IN GREEK MEDICINE

Whenever it was written, the vow to refer a patient to "practitioners of this activity" speaks of one way to minimize medical error. Surgery, unfortunately, is a fruitful place to explore the causes of, and ethical responses to, medical errors. The bold strokes of surgery, and the sharp change in a patient's condition before and after surgery, spotlight the surgeon's judgment and skill. The Greek physicians wrote about errors, their causes, and the use of error to improve medical practice.

The recording of medical errors and bad outcomes were natural observations by which physicians strove to improve medical practice. This forthright admission of an error, by the physician author of *Epidemic V*, illustrates the disclosure of error, its mortal effect, and the comment on the lesson that he learned:

> Autonomous in Omilus died on the sixteenth day from a head wound in midsummer. The stone, thrown by hand, hit him in the middle of the sutures on the front of the head. I was unaware that I should trephine because I did not notice that the sutures had the injury of the weapon, right on them, since it became obvious later.[31]

Four centuries later, the Roman writer Celsus said that this "sincere confession of the truth befits a great mind which will still be ready to accept many responsibilities, and especially in performing the task of handing down knowledge for the advantage of posterity that no one else may be deceived again by what has deceived him."[32] The medical book *Diseases I* identifies four types of errors: 1) failing to tell the patient the prognosis, good or unfavorable; 2) incorrect physical exams; 3) incorrect treatment; and 4) incorrect prognoses.[33] A careful review of case records in the various texts finds an even richer classification of pharmaceutical, surgical, and counseling errors (see Table 9–2). Of course, not every error results in a bad outcome, but a bad outcome does raise the specter of error.

The records of bad outcomes were both naturalistic observations of disease and used to evaluate and apportion culpability for that result between the physician, patient, or the disease itself. All the combinations were explored. This example from *Affections* discusses the relative role of the physician versus the disease in causing a bad outcome:

TABLE 9.2. Examples of Kinds of Medical Errors from Greek Medical Texts

Type of Error	Example
A physician's lack of technical skill	Tychon, at the siege of Datum, was struck in the chest by a catapult.... The physician who removed the wood seemed to me to leave the iron in at the diaphragm.[67] At Omilus, a young girl of about twelve years died in midsummer from a wound in the head.... Someone hit her with a door and crushed and shattered her skull. This was recognized properly as needing trephination. It was trephined, but not sufficiently.[68]
A physician's lack of experience	Nor indeed do I see that physicians are experienced in the proper way to distinguish the kind of weakness that occurs in disease, whether it be caused by starving, or by some other irritations, or by pain, or by the acuteness of the disease ... and that through a knowledge of such things brings safety and ignorance brings death.[69] [With regard to correcting a dislocation] It is not enough to know the art in theory only, but by familiar practice.[70]
A physician's undue confidence in a theory	[With regard to dislocated shoulders] Others have theories and practice the reverse of what is appropriate.[71]
A physician's innovative experiment	I once tried to make extension of the back [by an innovative treatment] ... but my attempt was not a success.... I relate this on purpose: for those things also give good instruction which after trial show themselves failures, and show why they failed.[72]
A physician's lack of understanding of either what is a natural or a healthy norm	The practitioner made him hold [and then splinted his injured arm] as the archers do.... This gave an appearance of wisdom to his course and practice but he had forgotten the other arts and all those things which are executed by strength or artifice, not knowing that the natural position varies in one and another....[73]

A physician's lack of knowledge when advising a patient	So there is radical ignorance among both those who use unstrained gruel and those who use only the juice. . . . All these things are strong testimony that physicians do not correctly guide their patients in the matter of regimen.[74]
A physician trying to impress a patient	If the nose is broken . . . those who delight in fine bandaging without judgment do more damage than usual . . . those who devote themselves to a foolish parade of manual skill are especially delighted to find a fractured nose to bandage. The result is that the practitioner rejoices and the patient is pleased for one or two days; afterwards the patient soon has enough of it for the burden is tiresome; and as for the practitioner, he is satisfied with showing that he knows how to apply complicated nasal bandages.[75]
A physician who errs by practicing to build a public reputation	What you should put first in all the practice of our art is how to make the patient well and if he can be made well in many ways, one should choose the least troublesome. This is more honorable and more in accord with the art for anyone who is not covetous of the false coin of popular advertisement.[76]
A physician who complies with a patient's demand for the wrong therapy	[Applying a hollow splint to a broken leg:] The vulgar have greater faith in it, and the practitioner will be more free from blame if a hollow splint is applied though it is rather bad practice.[77]
A lay healer's mistreatment	The boy from Metrophantus' house, wounded in the head with a potsherd by another child, became feverish after twelve days had passed. The explanation: the woman who washed the wound rubbed the area around it and it took a chill.[78]

Let nothing bad be added by the person treating—rather let the evils resulting from the diseases suffice. . . . If, when the physician treats correctly, the patient is overcome by the magnitude of the disease, this is not the physician's fault. But if, when the physician treats incorrectly or out of ignorance, the patient is overcome, it is his fault.[34]

In this passage from *Epidemics V*, a defensive physician argues that the surgery was done correctly even though the patient died.

Hippocomus, son of Palamedes in Larissa, eleven years old, was struck on the forehead above the right eye by a horse. The bone did not seem sound and a little blood spurted out of it. He was trephined extensively down to the bone surface. And he was cured despite the bone, which was already festering. He became fevered. . . . His eyes swelled, and his face. . . . The [surgical] wound was not responsible for his problems.[35]

This passage from *The Art* argues that sometimes a patient rather than the physician should be held culpable for an avoidable death.

Surely it is much more likely that the physician gives proper orders, which the patient not unnaturally is unable to follow; and not following them, he meets with death, the cause of which illogical reasoners attribute to the innocent, allowing the guilty to go free.[36]

One has to admit that the metaphor that likens a deceased, non-compliant patient to a guilty person who goes free is quite a bit of physicianly *chutzpah*. But Greek medicine does have its resemblances to the medicine of today.

Greek attention to the blameworthiness for bad outcomes continues to this day. Deaths from cancer spur research to improve treatments for cancer and of patient behaviors that increase the chances of getting cancer. Attributing a bad outcome to selecting a drug or to administering 10 milligrams of a drug when 10 micrograms was the correct dose spurs work on quality-improvement programs, and courses in physician handwriting. Finding that patients do not always take therapy is leading to work to improve patient education, simplify drug regimens, alleviate barriers to health care, and develop therapies with fewer side effects. Assigning culpability is key to the success or failure of lawsuits against physicians or tobacco companies.

* * *

CASE 9.1 A nurse, Sarah Jefferson, discovered the elderly, disabled Ms. Alice Rundell trapped and suffocated in the space between the mattress and the bedrails of her nursing home bed. For several months, Ms. Rundell, a small woman with Alzheimer's disease, had been moving restlessly in her bed. Twice in the month before she died, the nurses and aides had found her in the space between her mattress and rails. For five years before her death, professional journals and government alerts had been sent to nursing homes describing the hazard of suffocation between the rails and mattress, especially for persons like Ms. Rundell.

The Director of Nursing ordered Nurse Jefferson to tell the family that Ms. Rundell had died in her sleep. Ms. Jefferson refused to do so. She overheard the nursing supervisor tell Ms. Rundell's daughter that her mother had died peacefully in her sleep. The Director of Nursing and the administrator instructed Ms. Jefferson to not record details about the death in the medical record. The Director of Nursing also told staff not to discuss the death with staff in other parts of the facility. The physician knew about the circumstances of the death but remained silent.

Two days after the death, the mortician told relatives that the police were investigating a tip that Ms. Rundell had suffocated. As the family assembled at the church for the funeral, the coroner demanded the body for an autopsy. The funeral service proceeded with an empty casket. The coroner concluded that Ms. Rundell had suffocated in the bed equipment. The supervising nurses and the administrator all denied knowing about the duty to report unusual deaths to the medical examiner. The family sued the nursing home.[37]

Physicians and other health professionals study medical error today for the same reasons that the Greeks did: to improve medical care and to apportion responsibility for bad outcomes. Medical errors are the eighth most common cause of death in the United States, causing between 45,000 and 100,000 deaths per year.[38] This toll outranks AIDS, breast cancer, and even traffic accidents. Law, medicine, and ethics have each proposed ways to address this problem.[39] They include promoting research into why errors occur and mandating the reporting of adverse events so that they can be understood. Health-care professionals are taught about the types of errors that are most likely to occur in their settings. At "Morbidity and Mortality" conferences, health professionals frankly discuss and learn from their errors.[40] Quality improvement programs are implemented to change health-care institutions in ways that make errors less likely. Finally, punitive sanctions in the form of fines and lawsuits are imposed to promote attention to reducing bad outcomes.

These mechanisms failed Ms. Rundell. There is scant research on medical error in nursing homes. Bedrails were introduced without any research to show that they improved patient care or how to reduce the spaces in which a small person like Ms. Rundell could become trapped. There was no education on this kind of entrapment until 1996, forty years after the first deaths were reported. Nursing homes and manufacturers failed to report deaths in bedrails, thereby hindering public recognition of this problem. Ms. Rundell's providers expressed surprise when they learned the frequency of these kinds of accidents. Lawsuits and fines against nursing homes are rare and small compared to the severity of the injury. It is however, the concealment of the error from Ms. Rundell's family that takes this discussion back to ancient Greece.

What might ancient Greek physicians have had to say about Ms. Rundell? As we have seen, Greek writings supported sharing information in the medical community about medical errors in order to improve medical practice. The ethic is old, even if using coroners to investigate deaths, government agencies to compile and act on reports of adverse medical events, and medical boards to investigate incompetent physicians are new. The Greek physicians recognized, as we do, that errors are a form of data that should be used to improve medicine. As the author of *The Art* put it:

> Mistakes, no less than benefits, witness to the existence of the art and science; for what benefited did so because correctly administered, and what harmed did so because incorrectly administered.[41]

There is a notable difference, however, between how Greek physicians handled medical error and medical ethics for such events today. None of the dozens of accounts of errors in the ancient Greek texts advocates or illustrates telling a patient or a relative about an error.

Greek physicians were sensitive about the effect of error on their professional reputation. They also feared being unfairly accused of error:

> If a physician gives anything to a woman in childbed for the pain in her belly and she becomes worse or even dies, the physician will be blamed. Generally speaking, people blame the physician, in diseases and wounds, for the evils that follow of necessity other evils.[42]

Today, physicians' organizations, medical ethicists, and malpractice defense lawyers increasingly urge physicians to disclose medical errors to patients or their relatives.[43] This practice is controversial. Physicians and health facility administrators fear that such disclosures will lead to malpractice lawsuits, regulatory fines, and higher insurance premiums. They are also concerned that disclosing an error will result in bad publicity, loss of patients, and undue criticism of respected clinicians.[44]

Such fears must be put in context.[45] Concealing errors undermines public trust in health care, and, if uncovered, makes relatives or patients angry and more inclined to sue for very large sums.[46] When a court learns that a clinician has concealed an error by tampering with a medical record, it may impose major penalties for tampering with the evidence or even make a summary verdict against the clinician.[47] In the largest sense, concealing errors from patients and families fosters a destructive cynicism about health care that weakens physicians', nurses', and nurse's aides' respect for their work and impedes the larger effort to improve the quality of the health-care system. Generally, open communication decreases the chance of malpractice suits.[48] The duty to inform patients or their relatives of medical errors is a new step in the evolution of medical ethics, one that builds on the foundations of the ethics of error that the Greek physicians laid.

NOTES

1. *See In the Surgery; On the Diseases of Women I:70; Mochlicon; On Fractures; Head Wounds; Haemorrhoids.*

2. *Physician* 2,14.

3. Wangensteen and Wangensteen 313, 306.

4. Wangensteen and Wangensteen 9, 188, 193, 199.

5. Wangensteen and Wangensteen 17–18. One exception is bloodletting. Transverse incisions across vessels at various locations are described in countless sections of the texts. *Diseases III*:10 (nipples), *Diseases III*:7 ("his arms, his nose, his tongue and in fact, all over"); *Internal Affections* 4, 28,37, *Ulcers*:26.

6. Veatch [1981] 93.

7. *Internal Affections* 14.

8. Murphy 22. *Internal Affections* 15 and 17 describe surgery for different renal diseases that could well be perinephric hematomas and abscesses, respectively.

9. Littré 1844, 618 (Miles translation.) Nittis (op. cit.) agrees with the castration hypothesis and discusses speculation that necrosis of the testicles was a common complication of damaging blood vessels around the neck of the bladder. It seems very un-

likely that the urethral catheterization approach described in the ancient Greek treatise *Diseases I* would cause testicular ischemia, given the blood supply to the testis though it is possible that the post-operative care, such as bandages, could cause testicular ischemia. Cutting around the bladder neck was part of the surgical procedure developed by Ammonius that could have caused impotence.

10. They record a variety of observations on the cervix and uterus. *Epidemics* 2.2.7 describes a swelling of the testicle, but the management is not discussed.

11. See Chapter 3 for a discussion of Edelstein's controversial solution.

12. Veatch (1981) 93.

13. Kass 235–6.

14. Murphy 18–33.

15. Kass 232.

16. *Fractures, Mochlicon, Epidemics V* and *Epidemics VII* appear to have been written by persons with experience in military trauma.

17. Arguments for a prudent proportionality between treatment and outcome are not arguments against surgery. Take, for example, "Give to each disease according to its nature: in weak diseases give medications by nature weak, in strong diseases by nature strong" (*Places in Man* 45). Or, in referring to various ways to fix a dislocated shoulder, "You should use the most powerful one when you see the strongest need, and the method that will be described last will be the most powerful" (*On Joints I*). Or, "When the disease is very acute, it is essential to employ a regimen of extreme strictness . . . relax the strictness accordingly as the disease is milder" (*Aphorisms I:7*).

18. "Tis not a skillful leech who mumbles charms over ills that need the knife." (Sophocles. *Ajax* 581–2). Gorgias: "I have often, along with my brother and with other physicians, visited one of their patients who refused to drink his medicine or submit to the surgeon's knife or cautery, and when the doctor was unable to persuade them, I did so not by other art but rhetoric." Plato. *Gorgias* 456b. See also Plato: *Protagoras* 354; *Statesman* 293b; *Statesman* 298a–b.

19. For example, "to incise the anus, to amputate from it, to lift it by sewing, to cauterize it, or to remove something from it by putrefaction—these seem to be dangerous, but in fact, will do no harm." *Haemorrhoids* 2.

20. Withington 90–1. Majno 355. Though the Greeks recognized the importance of developing skills for specialized or dangerous procedures, this is not the same thing as dividing the field into surgeons and internists and "healthy lifestyle consultants" as apparently happened during the Roman era. For example, the following passage is a Greek description of how the specialized procedures for removing large foreign bodies requires skills that an ordinary physician surgeon would not have. "Related to this is the surgery of wounds . . .which concerns the extraction of missiles. In city practice experience of these is but little, for rarely even in a whole lifetime are there civil or

military combats. . . . Thus, the person intending to practice this kind of surgery must serve in the army, and accompany it on expeditions abroad; for in this way he would become experienced in this practice. . . . Only someone who is knowledgeable about these signs can properly put his hand to the task" (*Physician 14*). Greek surgeons practiced multimodal therapies. *Fractures*, for example, is the quintessential text for orthopedic surgery. It gives these instructions for treatment after realigning (reducing) an open fracture of the arm or leg: "After reduction one should give a mild dose of hellebore . . . Apply nothing cold and prescribe entire abstinence from solid food. . . . If he is of a bilious nature give him a little aromatic honeycomb in water, but if not, use water as a beverage . . . then return by a regular gradation to ordinary diet" (*Fractures XXXVI*).

21. Withington (Hippocrates [1928]xviii); Jones (Hippocrates [1923a]296 n2).

22. Celsus. *On Medicine V:1, VII:1*.

23. Celsus. *De Med.VII:26*. Murphy 23.

24. Nittis S. The authorship and probable date of the Hippocratic Oath. Bull Hist Med 1940;8:1012–21. See also Jouanna 401–2 and Carrick 85–6, 99–100.

25. The *Oath* is a composite document in that it includes the oath and the indenturing contract. (Jones in Hippocrates [1923a] 292). See also Jouanna 47. See Chapter 3 for a brief discussion of corruption of the treatises. Most the individual books of treatises discuss the problems of corrupted texts as well.

26. Nutton V. What's in an oath? J Roy Coll Phys in London 1995;29:518–24.

27. In personal correspondence, Vivian Nutton believes that the insertion hypothesis is possible but unlikely. He surmises that the cutting passage may refer to some kind of bloodletting taboo, but he is not aware of any citation of a fragment of the *Oath* with the surgical passage that predates the Roman era.

28. "The μήν in οὐδέ μήν λιθιώνας will strike scholars as strange." Jones in Hippocrates [1923a] 296 n2.

29. In this way, this passage also disrupts the stanzaic organization of the *Oath*'s middle section that I proposed in the introduction to Part II.

30. Another possibility would be the neo-Pythagoreans who emerged in the first century BCE after three hundred years of silence after the Pythagorean school. Being interested in science and mysticism, they would have been interested in the *Oath* and, if they were aware of it, may have been inclined to amend it to argue for a nonsurgical medicine. If the neo-Pythagoreans did amend the *Oath* by inserting this passage, it seems odd that they did not go further to make the Oath to conform to their views by removing the pessary restriction from the passage on abortion and altering the last section, which speaks about the human accountability of medicine, an un-Pythagorean viewpoint.

31. *Epidemics 5:27*.

32. Celsus. *De Medicina IV:5.*

33. *Diseases I:6.*

34. *Affections 13.*

35. *Epidemics 5:16.*

36. *The Art VII.*

37. Miles SH. Concealing accidental nursing home deaths. Health Care Ethics Committee Forum 2002;14:224–34.

38. Committee 2000.

39. Pinkus RL. Mistakes as a social construct: A historical approach. Kennedy Inst Ethics J 2001;11:117–33.

40. Bosk.

41. *The Art V.*

42. *Diseases I:8.*

43. Rosner F, Berger JT, Kark P, et al. Disclosure and prevention of medical errors. Arch Intern Med 2000;160:2089–92.

44. Pietro DA, Shavitz L, Smith RA, Auerbach BS. Detecting and reporting medical errors: Why the dilemma? BMJ 2000;320(7237):794–6. Anonymous. Five times: Coincidence or something more serious? BMJ 1998;316(7146):1736–7.

45. Kapp MB. Medical error vs. malpractice. DePaul J Health Care Law 1997;1: 751–72.

46. Witman AB, Park DM, Hardin S. How do patients want physicians to handle mistakes? A survey of internal medicine patients in an academic setting. Arch Intern Med 1996;156:2265–9.

47. Gilbert JL, Whitworth RL, Ollanik SA, Hare FH. Evidence destruction—legal consequences of spoilation of records. Legal Medicine 1994:181–200.

48. Levinson W, Roter DL, Mullooly JP, et al. Physician–patient communication. The relationship with malpractice claims among primary care physicians and surgeons. JAMA 1997;277:553–9.

49. *Places in Man 32; Epidemics 4:11; Epidemics 5:27; Epidemics 5:28; Epidemics 5:16; On Head Wounds 12–15.*

50. *Epidemics 7:35; Epidemics 5:15.*

51. *Head Wounds 12–20.*

52. *Physician 14.*

53. Wangensteen and Wangensteen 40.

54. Wangensteen and Wangensteen 305.

55. *Internal Affections 9; Diseases III:16;* Wangensteen and Wangensteen 9, 188, 193, 199.

56. *Epidemics 5:26; Internal Affections 9.*

57. *Haemorrhoids 2; Regimen in Acute Disease (Appendix) a62.*

58. *Internal Affections* 14, 15, 17. See text on stones.

59. *Diseases* I:6. Various parsings of this passage are offered. Potter translates it as "surgically incorrect are the following: [list] . . . not to be able to succeed in inserting a tube into the bladder; not to recognize that there is a stone in the bladder; . . ." (Hippocrates [1988]). Nitis translates this as "introducing a catheter, not to be able to reach the bladder or reaching it, not to be able to locate the stone." (Nittis S. The Hippocratic Oath in reference to lithotomy. Bull Hist Med 1939;7:719–28.) Littré translates it as: "In surgery, it is a blunder to be unable to catheterize, arrive in the bladder and once there to be unaware of the presence of a stone." (Littré 1844, 616. [Miles translation.]) It seems fair to assume as Nittis and Littré do that this passage refers to passing a device along the urethra to remove a bladder stone.

60. *Internal Affections* 23.

61. *Internal Affections* 24.

62. *Internal Affections* 41.

63. *Places in Man* 25; *Internal Affections* 23.

64. *On the Diseases of Women* I:70 in Hanson, op. cit., 1991.

65. *Diseases* II: 33,35.

66. *Affections* 4.

67. *Epidemics* 7:121.

68. *Epidemics* 5:28.

69. *Regimen in Acute Disease* XLIII (Hippocrates [1950]).

70. *Joints* X.

71. *Joints* XI.

72. *Joints* XLVII.

73. *Fractures* II.

74. *Regimen in Acute Diseases* XL–XLI.

75. *Joints* XXXV.

76. *Joints* LXXVIII. See also the anecdote on dropping patients to straighten a spine from *On Joints* 42 (quoted in Chapter 11).

77. *Fractures* XVI.

78. *Epidemics* 4:11.

10

CONSENT AND TRUTH-TELLING

INTO AS MANY HOUSES AS I MAY ENTER, I WILL GO FOR THE
BENEFIT OF THE ILL . . .

This passage contains two elements, a shift of scene ("Into as many houses as
I may enter"), and a statement of the purpose of the clinical encounter ("I will
go for the benefit of the ill"). As noted in the introduction to Part II, "I enter"
is the only time that the *Oath* uses verbs that are not part of a moral vow or
assessments; as such, this verb signals a shift in moral sphere, specifically to
the house.

ENTERING THE HOUSE

This entering of the house appears to represent the physician's movement into
the private and personal sphere of the patient and his or her family. Three lines
of evidence support this reading. First, the *Oath* uses the feminine form of the
word for house, *oikia*. Some scholars believe that the masculine form had a
narrower connotation, referring simply to a dwelling structure. The feminine
form may have denoted the house as a social space.[1] If this selection of gender
was intended and was meaningful in this manner, then the *Oath* is emphasiz-
ing that the clinical encounter morally takes place in the patient's private and
familial space even when the physician treats the patient in a public location.

The medical treatises and other historical documents describe medical care taking place in public locations, somewhat akin to unsecluded clinics and partly for advertising purposes. Second, once the house is entered, the next two passages identify specific forms of injustice, which are defined as transgressions against the private sphere of life: sexual relations that would only be possible in intimate and enclosed space of a house, and revealing information from the patient's private world to the outside world. Third, once this private sphere is entered, the *Oath* refers to patients with the recognizably personal attributes of gender and social status. For these reasons, the *Oath* uses *house* to refer to more than a physical house or enclosed structure. Rather, it is a social space in which various people live, where intimacy is possible and can be violated, and where confidences that must not be revealed are disclosed.

PATERNALISM

The physician enters the patient's private world vowing to "go for the benefit of the ill." Ancient physicians seemed to understand this aim of medicine much as we do. As the author of *Art* puts it, "I would define medicine as the complete removal of the distress of the sick, the alleviation of the more violent diseases."[2] It is noteworthy that this focus on restoring health does not encompass the explicit aim of prolonging life, one of the most ardent aims of modern medicine.[3] This book will not focus on the therapies these physicians used; rather, it focuses on ethics, and in this case, on how the conduct of the physician–patient relationship was understood as benefiting the ill. Patient education, the frank disclosure of diagnoses, and informed consent to treatment are seen as modern prerequisites for a good physician–patient relationship and as ways to effectively engage the patient as a partner in treatment. Was it so in ancient Greece?

Modern medical ethicists, with the exception of Jonsen,[4] have tended to assess the physician–patient relationship in Greek medicine as paternalistic. Medical paternalism describes the practice in which a physician unilaterally decides to conceal information in order to coerce a patient into accepting a treatment or because of a mistaken belief that patients are generally psychologically harmed by bad news. As Veatch put it: "The old Hippocratic ethic saw the patient as a weak, debilitated, childlike victim, incapable of functioning as a real moral agent. [He went on to conclude with evident relief] . . . The Hippocratic ethic is dead."[5] Today, the requirement that a patient give "informed consent" to a medical interview, physical examination, and treatment is the centerpiece of clinical ethics. It is anchored on the principle of respect for the patient's autonomy and protected by law. If Veatch is correct, a moral chasm separates modern medical ethics from ancient Greece. There is little evidence, however, that Greek physicians either paternalistically withheld information or coercively misled patients to comply with treatment.

Critics of Greek clinical ethics often cite *Decorum* and *Precepts* to make the case for Greek medical paternalism.[6] These two works, written centuries after the *Oath*, portray a much more patrician physician than is depicted in the medical literature of the *Oath's* time. The most frequently cited passage is from *Decorum*:[7]

> Perform these duties calmly and adroitly, concealing most things from the patient while you are attending to him. Give necessary orders with cheerfulness and serenity, turning his attention away from what is being done to him; sometimes reprove sharply and emphatically . . . revealing nothing of the patient's future or present condition.[8]

Scholars of ancient Greece have long criticized *Decorum*. Jones, whose translation is the most widely used, notes that it appears to have been written in the early Christian era and says that the author had "an imperfect knowledge of Greek." He adds that "there is something unnatural and fantastic about certain parts of it; one might say that the obscurity was apparently intentional."[9] Temkin takes a similarly dim view, asserting that, "The text of *Decorum* and *Precepts* is badly corrupted and the interpretation of many passages relies on conjecture."[10] Thus, the most widely cited textual evidence of Greek medical paternalism does not seem to be representative of ancient Greece.

PERSUASION

Greek physicians had to persuade patients to seek them out, to accept recommendations, and to pay for services.[11] They faced competition from herbalists, traditional healers, and temple healers. Temple healers had a competitive advantage in being able to explain their failures as due to an overpowering curse, while physicians could only explain their failures by pleading the imperfection of their new science. Greek patients had various opportunities to observe a physician before choosing to engage his services. Physicians lectured on health to public gatherings.[12] Relatives and public spectators watched as doctors made prognoses and practiced surgery.[13] Physicians who applied to be city-physicians submitted to public questioning. As Plato acerbically noted, a charlatan who was more artful at persuading lay people of his medical prowess had an advantage over a more competent, but less rhetorically skilled, physician.[14] The intensity of this public competition is reflected in extensive medical writings about how to enhance one's reputation and build a successful practice.

This competition also led physicians to bemoan the practices of their competitors. They complained about prognostic show-offs:

[T]here are reports of physicians making frequent true and marvelous predictions, predictions such as I have never made myself . . . [such as] to foretell in merchants and adventurers death to some, madness to others, and other diseases to others.[15]

They denounced quackery, as in this acid comment about healers who built reputations by dropping suspended persons from ladders to straighten curved spines:

the practitioners who use this method are chiefly those who want to make the vulgar herd gape, for to such it seems marvelous to see a man suspended or shaken or treated in such ways; and they always applaud these performances, never troubling themselves about the result of the operation, whether good or bad.[16]

They decried showmanship in gaudy equipment:

The physician should avoid the use of bronze, except for his instruments, for the use of such gear seems to me to be nothing but vulgar ostentation.[17]

They remonstrated against physicians who pandered to patients by practicing bad medicine (see Table 9.2). It would be interesting to know what they would have said about modern cosmetic surgeons who advertise their skill with depictions of the Greek goddess, Aphrodite. All in all, the ancient Greek physicians practiced in a competitive market place in which they had many kinds of opportunities to promote their skill, in which there were competitive abuses, and in which a head of household voluntarily invited a physician to care for his family and slaves.

OPENING THE PHYSICIAN–PATIENT CONVERSATION

The role of paternalism in the medical ethics of ancient Greece is not contradicted merely by the finding that a physician was freely chosen. The paternalism issue simply unfolds to a deeper level. Did ancient physicians tell patients the truth about their diagnoses, prognoses, and the nature of treatments? Did the physician work for the patient's benefit by fostering an informed and consenting partnership with the patient? From a social perspective, the image of physicians' haughtily dictating orders to Greek freemen seems at odds with the egalitarianism of Greek culture. Plato, writing at the time the *Oath* was written, extensively discusses the voluntary and informed relationship between physicians and patients.[18] More specifically, the medical treatises of the *Oath's* time depict an attractive model for physician–patient communication and securing consent. As the first of the *Aphorisms* pointedly says: "The physician must be ready, not only to do his duty himself, but also to secure the cooperation of the patient."[19] How did Greek physicians secure the patient's cooperation with the medical interview, examination, and treatment?

The physician–patient conversation described in Greek texts began by listening to the patient. Skill in this task was not taken to be self-evident. The following passage from a gynecological treatise instructed physicians on how to listen to women:

> You cannot disregard what women say about childbearing. For they are talking about what they know and are always inquiring about. . . . It is the women who make the judgments and who award the prize. . . . [20]

This passage reaffirms the importance of listening to what a woman had to say.

> Sometimes diseases become incurable for women who do not learn why they are sick before the doctor has been correctly taught by the sick woman why she is sick. For women are ashamed to tell even if they know and they suppose that it is a disgrace, because of their inexperience and lack of knowledge. At the same time the doctors also make mistakes by not learning the apparent cause through

accurate questioning, but they proceed to heal as though they were dealing with men's diseases.[21]

The gendered assumptions in this passage are noteworthy. On one hand, it depicts women as reticent, embarrassed to speak, and uninformed. On the other hand, physicians are depicted as assuming that women's diseases are just like men's and not giving proper weight to women's accounts of their symptoms, a critique of male physicians that is too often true today.

The aim of listening to a patient was to discern a clinical syndrome. Recognition of syndromic patterns served as the basis for recommending a treatment even though the underlying pathophysiology or etiology of the disorder was unknown. Trauma and pregnancy were the only conditions with self-evident causes. The discovery of germs, genes, and pathophysiology lay in the distant future. There were no lab tests, scans, stethoscopes, or thermometers. Not surprisingly, syndromic recognition is difficult to practice. Various diseases present the same signs and symptoms. For example, many diseases have the syndrome of a sense of warmth, muscle aches, fatigue, and shortness of breath on exertion. The author of *Prognosis* despaired of naming diseases at all: "There is no point in seeking the name of any disease [for all] may be recognized by the same signs."[22] This, for example, is a syndromic description of the signs and prognosis of the bacterial disease that we call tetanus: "If in a person suffering from a fever, the neck be suddenly twisted round and swallowing becomes almost impossible though there is no swelling, then he will die."[23]

To complicate matters further, the same disease will manifest itself and progress differently in different people. One person may die of pneumonia while another lives. To reduce the inherent imprecision of syndromic diagnosis, Greek physicians performed detailed histories and examinations. They noted the setting: climate, weather, and season. The patient's age, gender, habits, household, diet, appetite, and thirst were important factors. The physician noted the fluency of speech, rationality of thought, mood, sleep, dreams, weeping, and laughing. Symptoms such as nausea, the location and severity of pain, occurrence of chills, coughs, sneezes, shivers, chills, hiccoughs, rigors, convulsions, nosebleeds, changes in menstruation, or failing vision or hearing were recorded. Behaviors such as plucking hair, scratching, twitches, speechlessness, belching, and flatulence were important. The physical examination paid attention to fever, patterns of breathing, paralysis, the color of the extremities, abnormal anatomy, pain on palpation, and the location and temperature of sweat. Stools, urine, sputum, and vomit were described.[24] Even so, this comprehensive evaluation was often insufficient to assess a patient's condition without one important additional observation: the course of the disease over time.

Physicians observed the temporal course of the illness, including the periodicity or irregularity of the waxing and waning of various signs and symptoms. Greek physicians needed time to observe the trajectory of a syndrome in order to make a prognosis. "Anyone who is to make a correct forecast of a patient's recovery or death, or the length of his illness, must be thoroughly acquainted with the signs and form his judgment by estimating their influence on one another."[25] Here is an example of how "time" enabled a physician to make an accurate prognosis in a person with pneumonia and pleurisy:

> [S]hould the empyema begin from sputum of this character when the disease has reached the seventh day, the patient may be expected to die on the fourteenth day unless some good symptoms happen to him. The good symptoms are these [a long list of indicators of a strong individual resistance to the disease]. If all these symptoms supervene, the patient will not die; if some, but not all, supervene, the patients will die after living for longer than fourteen days. . . . You must take into account both the good signs and the bad that occur and from them make your predictions: for in this way you will prophesy aright.[26]

Observations over time enabled a physician to make a prognosis of the nature of a disease and whether it would end in recovery, disability, or death. "Brilliant and effective forecasts are made by distinguishing the way, manner and time in which each case will end, either it takes the turn to recover or to incurability."[27] The time it took to arrive at syndromic prognosis posed an ethical problem for the physician's conversation with the patient. When, if ever, should the patient be told the prognosis?

DISCLOSING THE PROGNOSIS

Some scholars misread cautions to take time to observe the course of an illness as meaning that the physician should conceal or withhold a prognosis. This conclusion abuses the sense of passages from various Greek books. Acknowledging the difficulty of making a prognosis is not the same thing as saying that one should not disclose a prognosis. Thus, such examples as, "In the case of acute diseases, to predict either death or recovery is not quite safe [or not at all safe],"[28] or "[It] is not safe to make an advance statement before the disease is settled"[29] may not without corroborating evidence be taken as endorsing a paternalistic silence. That evidence, as we shall see, runs the other way. The precaution of taking time to observe the course of illness commends the development of an accurate prognosis much like the way a modern physician waits for the results of a biopsy before telling a patient the extent or grade or origin of a cancer. As the author of *Prorrhetic II* cautions, prognosis "is indeed possible [but] . . . I advise you to be as cautious as possible . . . in [predicting death, madness, or healing]. . . . When you are successful in making a prediction you will be admired by the patient you are tending, but when you go wrong you will not only be subject to hatred, but perhaps even be thought mad."[30]

The disclosure of the prognosis to the patient and to the patient's family benefited the patient and the physician. Disclosing the prognosis was fundamental to securing the collaboration of the patient with treatment. *Affections*, a treatise on pathophysiology, recommends telling patients what medicine can offer:

> Any man who is intelligent must, on considering that health is of the utmost value to human beings, have the personal understanding necessary to help himself in diseases, and be able to understand and to judge what physicians say and what they administer to his body, being versed in each of these matters to a degree reasonable for a layman.[31]

This admonition to speak plainly is repeatedly emphasized. As the author of *On Ancient Medicine* put it, "if anyone departs from what is popular knowledge and does not make himself intelligible to his audience, he is not being practical."[32] A forthright and ongoing dialogue also addressed issues relating to the risks of not following the physician's recommendation. As *Prorrhetic II* puts it, "the physician should indicate whatever is abnormal; for evils that arise as a result of noncompliance will be revealed as such, since the shortness of breath and the rest of the symptoms will cease on the following day, if they arose only because of a dietary mistake."[33] Finally, open disclosure of a prognosis directly benefited the physician's business.

> [If a physician] is able to tell his patients . . . not only about their past and present symptoms, but also tell them what is going to happen as well as to fill in the details they have omitted, he will increase his reputation . . . and people will have no

qualms in putting themselves under his care. Moreover, he will better be able to effect a cure. . . .[34]

In short, Greek medical works recommended disclosing the prognosis to benefit the patient and the physician.

The Greek physicians repeatedly said that bad news, like good, should be disclosed. For example, the author of *Diseases I* says that it is

> incorrect to say that a disease is different from what it really is, to say that a major disease is minor, or to say that a minor disease is major; not to tell a patient that is going to survive that he will survive, not to tell a patient about to die that he will die, . . . [or not] to say that what cannot be cured will be cured.[35]

The author of *On Head Wounds* has similar advice:

> When a patient is likely to die from his head wounds and cannot recover his health or be saved, it is by means of the following signs, then you must make the diagnosis that he is going to die and predict what is going to be.[36]

This is one example of what the sequence of syndromic recognition and disclosing a dire prognosis looked like:

> The commander of the large ship: the anchor crushed his forefinger, the bone below it on the right hand. Inflammation developed, gangrene. . . . Part of the finger fell away. . . . After that, problems with the tongue, he said he could not articulate anything. Prediction made that opisthonis [the lethal climax of tetanus] would come. His jaws became fixed together, then it went to the neck, on the third day he was entirely convulsed backward, with sweating. On the sixth day after the prediction, he died.[37]

Langholf, a modern scholar of ancient Greece, says that good and bad prognoses were to be disclosed because medical prognostication was respected as a secular analogue of divination, in which Greeks sought favorable and unfavorable prophesies on both medical and nonmedical affairs.[38]

The medical records of ancient Greece do not show paternalistic physicians. Patients, or at least the heads of households, chose the physician from among many healers in an intensely competitive environment. The physician did a complete medical history that could only be done with the patient's cooperation. Greek physicians saw such forthrightness as serving the patient's and the physician's interests. The patient and family were told of the prognosis as part of securing their cooperation with the recommended therapy, to enhance the physician's reputation, and to exempt the physician from being blamed for an unanticipated death. Information was not withheld to coerce patients to accept treatment.

*   *   *

CASE 10.1 Carl Swenson, an elderly man, was admitted to the hospital after he suffered a cardiac arrest. He had collapsed against the inside of the bedroom door at his home. His wife was in the hall outside the bedroom and could not push the door open. Twenty minutes later paramedics pushed their way in and started resuscitation that restored little more than a heartbeat. He was unconscious when admitted to a county hospital. His dilated pupils did not contract to a bright light. He did not blink when his eyes were touched or gag when the back of his throat was rubbed with a tongue depressor.

Carl was loved by a large family, including his wife, siblings, grown children, and grandchildren. He showed no change as his family gathered at the hospital over the course of several hours. It became clear that he had virtually no chance for recovery of significant brain function. I told the family of the severity of the brain damage as the results of the various diagnostic tests became available. The family members agreed that Carl would not want his life sustained under such circumstances. They asked their pastor to come to the hospital.

The minister arrived several hours later. I asked the nurses to remove unneeded, bulky equipment, such as the bed warmer, to make it easier for Mr. Swenson's relatives to approach his bedside. The bedrails were lowered and the restraints were removed. A suction tube that passed through his nose to his stomach was taken out. The relatives would now be able to hold free hands and kiss his unobstructed face. Video monitors that pointlessly displayed electronic traces of pulse, blood pressure, and breathing, were turned off. A box of tissues was placed on the bed for the tears that would come. I told the relatives that I would stay to make sure that Mr. Swenson's needs were met after the respirator was removed.

The minister read from the Bible and led the family in prayers. "Heavenly Father, we thank you for the life of Carl, our husband, father, brother, and friend. During his life, we realize how often we have taken Your gift of breath for granted. As his spirit now joins you, we are mindful of how each breath and his life was your inspiration." Relatives offered testimonials or spoke to the unconscious man. Some family members went to a waiting room; others stayed in the room. I covered the respirator tube with a small towel and quickly removed it. Mr. Swenson's face was now unencumbered by devices. The relatives reassembled and took turns holding his hands, kissing him, and saying goodbyes. More prayers were said. Mr. Swenson died eight hours later.[39]

As we look back with a modern horror at ancient practices of cautery with hot irons or amputations without anesthesia, it is easy to assume that physicians must have deceived patients into accepting such treatments. Nonetheless, a laymann like Plato noted patients' willingness to undergo arduous treatments: "Why sir, when men freely go to the physician for a course of medicaments, must we imagine they do not know they will very soon be, for days together, in such a state of body that, were it to be permanent they would be sick of life . . . [yet] they go of their own motion, for the sake of subsequent benefits."[40] Given the centrality of informed consent documents in modern medicine, it is understandable how we have taken the *Oath's* silence about informed consent as commending a medical paternalism that we have abandoned with such documented vigor. Perhaps medical ethicists' pride in articulating "respect for patient autonomy" and advancing its position in medical practice has blinded them to considering whether this idea might have a longer tradition in medical ethics.

The view that ancient Greek physicians were silent medical paternalists does not allow us to learn much from that medical culture about talking with Mr. Swenson's family. The *Oath's* silence, however, on medical truth-telling is insufficient to establish the case that Greek physicians mislead or coerced patients. The *Oath* is not a comprehensive compilation of the medical ethics of its time. The ancient Greek medical treatises show that Greek physicians did disclose prognoses and viewed the education of patients as essential to securing their cooperation with therapies. So perhaps modern medicine should have taken a cue from Greece before modern law and medical ethics "rediscovered" informed consent and truth-telling. Perhaps the ancient physicians even now have a lesson to teach about truth-telling.

Twenty-five years ago, U.S. physicians generally withheld bad news for fear that it would cause a patient to despair. That clinical dishonesty was extraordinarily destructive. Patients eventually came to know that they were terminally ill, and the silence that the physician had created allowed mistrust, fear, and loneliness to settle over the relationships between the patient, relatives, and the physician.[41] Patients were deprived of information that they needed to put their affairs in order and to have meaningful conversations with loved ones.

Today, American physicians generally accept the advice to tell patients the name of their diagnosis, however grave it may be.

The ancient Greek physicians revealed a prognosis rather than a diagnosis to patients and families. Part of the reason for this was that they lacked a science of pathophysiology and diagnostic tools that would have enabled them to formulate a diagnosis. The distinction between *diagnosis* and *prognosis* is important for informed consent. Ironically, in modern times, the ascendant practice of disclosing diagnoses has been accompanied by declining attention to disclosing prognoses.[42] Consider the difference between these two hypothetical ways of disclosing a terminal illness: "You have a difficult-to-treat brain cancer called glioblastoma," or "You have a brain cancer called glioblastoma. Treatment is difficult. There is a fifty percent chance of dying in one year and a seventy-five percent chance of dying in two years." The latter disclosure gives the patient information for making life plans. Many physicians find it stressful and difficult to disclose a prognosis or to answer a patient's questions, "How long will I live?" or "What will my ensuing illness feel like?" Many physicians, even though they reveal a diagnosis, provide vague or deceptively optimistic answers to patients who ask about such matters.[43] Half of today's medical students watch as their teachers lie to patients.[44]

The Greek records emphasize the importance of disclosing the prognosis. Given the ancient Greek physicians' conviction that disclosing the patient's future was necessary to secure the patient's trust and cooperation, it likely that would disagree with modern physicians who believe that disclosing a diagnosis would be an adequate substitute for telling the patient what the diagnosis portends. So what would Greek physicians have made of my conversations with Mr. Swenson's relatives after his cardiac arrest? Their writings show that they would have recognized the importance of gathering information before making a prediction. Evidence suggests that they would have revealed the prognosis as a way to display skill, foster trust, and set reasonable expectations for treatment "for the benefit of the ill."

NOTES

1. Scholars take both sides on the evidence for this connotative difference. Pomeroy 21–36; Cohen (1991) 70–97.

2. *The Art* 1:8 (Trans. from Chadwick who calls it *"The Science of Medicine"*).

3. Amundsen DW. The physician's obligation to prolong life: A medical duty without classical roots. Hastings Cent Rep 1978(Aug):23-30.

4. Jonsen (2000) 1-12.

5. Veatch (1987) 4, 37, 169. Veatch elaborates on this paternalism of Hippocratic medicine in "Medical Oaths and Codes: Ethical Analysis" (Reich 1428).

6. These three works are the cornerstone for Pellegrino's supportive views of the benevolent paternalistic physician even as he acknowledges that this is no longer the ideal for our time. (Pellegrino ED. "Toward an Expanded Medical Ethic: The Hippocratic Oath Revisited," in Bulger 45-64. Pellegrino 20-1). Nutton offers a detailed discussion of the problem with modern bioethicists and the *Oath*, "Hippocratic Morality and Modern Medicine," in Flashar and Jouanna 31-63. See also Nutton V. "Healers in the Medical Market Place: Towards a Social History of Graeco-Roman Medicine," in Wear 15-29.

Some also point to the *Oath's* words "I will use treatments for the benefit of the ill according to *my ability and judgment*" as showing paternalistic inclination. This passage precedes the clinical encounter that begins with "entering of the house." The clinical ethic "I will go for the benefit of the ill" does not include the allegedly paternalistic personal pronouns.

7. See Reiser SJ. Words as scalpels: Transmitting evidence in the clinical dialogue. Annals Int Med 1980;92:837-42. Amundsen D. "The Physician–Patient Relationship" (Reich 1511). Faden and Beauchamp 61. Applebaum, Lidz, and Meisel (163) quote Katz (4-7) on this citation. It is the basis for a similar conclusion by Beauchamp and Childress (393). Veatch, who believes in the Hippocratic paternalism of the physician–patient conversation, refers to the *Decorum* several times but does not mention specific passages.

8. *Decorum*: XVI. (This passage from about the time of Jesus.)

9. Jones in Hippocrates (1923b) 269-70, 306-7.

10. Temkin 25, n42.

11. Lloyd ([1979] 86-98) has a detailed discussion of the physician–patient conversations.

12. Lloyd (1987) 88-108.

13. Jouanna 76-7; Lloyd (1979) 90-4; Lloyd (1991) 136-40; *Nature of Man I*.

14. Plato. *Gorgias 456:bc*.

15. *Prorrhetic II:1*.

16. *Joints XLII*.

17. *Physician 2*. See also *Physician 4* on showy bandages that do not promote healing.

18. Plato was a keen scholar of physicians and often discusses the need to inform a patient and secure the patient's consent. For example, "One who advises a sick man

living in a way that injures his health that he must first effect a reform in his way of living, must he not? And if the patient consents to such a reform, then he may admonish him on other points? If, however, the patient refuses, in my opinion it would be the act of a real man and a good physician to keep clear of advising such a man" (Plato. *Letters VII:330:d*).

Though Plato saw consent as necessary to the physician–patient relationship, the ability to secure consent was not necessarily the measure of a physician. Plato tells an expert in rhetoric, Gorgias, "I have often, along with my brother and with other physicians, visited one of their patients, who refused to drink his medicine or submit to the surgeon's knife or cautery, and when the doctor was unable to persuade them, I did so by not other art but rhetoric" (Plato. *Gorgias 456 a–b*.). In *Laws*, he notes that a physician who "for the most part attends free men . . . takes the patient and his family into his confidence. Thus, he learns something from the sufferer, and at the same time instructs the invalid to the best of his powers. He does not give his prescription until he has won the patient's support, and when he has done so, he steadily aims at producing complete restoration to health by persuading the sufferer into compliance." (Plato. *Laws 4.720:d*.). See also Plato. *Statesman 293b*.

19. *Aphorisms 1*.

20. *On the Seventh-Month Child 4.1*.

21. *Diseases of Women I:62* (Hippocrates [1975]).

22. *Prognosis 25* (Hippocrates [1950]).

23. *Aphorisms VII:59a* (Hippocrates [1950]).

24. Examples taken from *Epidemics I*.

25. *Prognosis 25* in Hippocrates (1950). Note that "incurability" can refer to a condition from which one will die, an irreversible disability, or a condition that is not amenable to further treatment (von Staden H. "Incurability and Hopelessness: The Hippocratic Corpus," in Potter, Maloney, and Desautels 75–112).

26. *Prognostic xv*.

27. *Joints LVIII*.

28. *Aphorisms II:xix*.

29. *Prorrhetic II:3*.

30. *Prorrhetic II:2* (Hippocrates [1950]).

31. *Affections 1*. Potter notes that this sentence is often misread as introducing a medical treatise that was written for laymen; in fact this treatise addresses physicians and contains advice on how to educate patients (Hippocrates [1988] 4).

32. *Tradition in Medicine 2* in Hippocrates (1950). See Lloyd (1979) 95.

33. *Prorrhetic II:3* (I have changed "disobedience" to the contemporary medical term of "noncompliance.") See, for example, the discussion of management of a broken collarbone in *Joints 14*.

34. *Prognosis 1* (Hippocrates [1950]).

35. *Diseases I:6.* Katz's misreads this passage as arguing for concealing information because he relies on a secondary source that took it out of context (Katz 6).

36. *On Head Wounds 12:19* (Hippocrates [1950]).

37. *Epidemics 5:74.*

38. Langholf 232–54.

39. Miles SH. "The Role of Physicians in Sacred End-of-Life Rituals in the ICU," in *Managing Death in the ICU: The Transition from Cure to Comfort.* eds. JR Curtis and GD Rubenfield. New York: Oxford University Press, 2000, 207–12.

40. Plato. *Laws I;646:c.*

41. Katz.

42. Christakis NA. The ellipsis of prognosis in modern medical thought. Soc Sci & Med 1997;44:301–15.

43. Christakis NA, Iwashyna TJ. Attitude and self-reported practice regarding prognostication in a national sample of internists. Arch Intern Med 1998;158:2389–95. Lamont EB, Christakis NA. Prognostic disclosure to patients with cancer near the end of life. Ann Intern Med 2001;134:1096–1105.

44. Feudtner C, Christakis DA, Christakis NA. Do clinical clerks suffer ethical erosion? Students' perceptions of their ethical environment and personal development. Acad Med 1994;69:670–9.

11

EXPLOITING PATIENTS

... WHILE BEING FAR FROM ALL VOLUNTARY AND DESTRUCTIVE
INJUSTICE, ESPECIALLY FROM SEXUAL ACTS BOTH UPON
WOMEN'S BODIES AND UPON MEN'S, BOTH OF THE FREE AND OF
THE SLAVES.

Medical ethicists simply accept the latter part of this passage as a disavowal of
sexual relations with patients. There is little scholarship on what this pledge
might have been saying in its own time.[1] It exceeded the standard set by Athenian law, which is not known to have forbidden voluntary sexual relations
between physicians and patients or members of a patient's household. The
passage did not give latitude to consensual or purchased sexual services. The
rigor of this vow may have partly reflected the fact that a guardian or head of
household who hired out the services of a free woman, girl, or boy for sexual
purposes could be charged with prostitution, a potentially capital offence.[2]
Thus, the allegation that a head of household had bartered a household
member's sexual services for a physician's services would be dangerous indeed.

Aside from the extreme criminal charge of procurement, this passage seems
most akin to ancient Greek civil rules of hospitality, *xenos*, that forbade guests to
have sex with a member of the household.[3] A guest who raped or seduced a free
female member of a household could be killed, beaten, or forced to pay monetary compensation to her male guardian. Though the norms of *xenos* did not

apply to tradespeople, different social standards imposed a comparable standard for behavior. Though a physician's visit was an act of commerce, the *Oath's* assertion that clinical care morally took place in the "house," regardless of where it physically took place, suggests that physicians viewed the ethics of clinical care as falling within the ethics of a guest relationship. It would have been useful to stand under the rules of *xenos* since this would have helped the public understand the ethics of the new profession, and this would have called for a greater intimacy in disclosure and greater assurances of secrecy than applied to encounters with tradespeople. If this is an accurate reading, this passage prohibited sexual relationships with any member of a patient's household and not simply with the patient. Furthermore, violating this passage would have been a transgression that dishonored the physician-guest as well as the individual members of the household and its name, for which the guardian was responsible.[4]

The concerns that led to this vow were perhaps illustrated by an account by Ctesius, a Greek physician of around 400 BCE (approximately the time when the *Oath* was written).[5] He was a physician to Persian royalty and wrote of a Persian princess, Amytis, who

> fell sick but not gravely so. Apollonides, a physician from Cos [the site of the medical school founded by Hippocrates], was quite taken with her. He told her that she could recover her health by having relations with men. His subterfuge succeeded and he became her lover but she did not fully yield to him. Then, he completely withdrew from her. As she died, Amytis told her mother to punish him. Her mother went to king Artoxerxes and told him of the relationship and how Apollonides had turned from Amytis after dishonoring and abusing her vows. The king gave the mother carte blanche to deal with the matter. She had Apollonides imprisoned and tortured for two months as his cries for mercy rang out. Then she entombed him alive.[6]

It is not clear that whoever wrote the *Oath* knew this story, and Ctesius was known to have embellished his stories. The snide mention of Apollonides' medical training at Cos may be explained by the fact that Ctesius was trained at the competing medical school on Cnidos. Cnidian alumnae may also have been responsible for libeling Hippocrates with the charge that he burned their library.

The physician not only disavows sexual acts with women, like Amytis, but also abjures sexual relations with men. Greek society accepted voluntary sexual relations between adult men and boys from about twelve to eighteen years old, though sexual relationships between adult men and young free girls were unacceptable. There was some ambivalence about these homosexual acts. The society expected post-adolescent men to live as heterosexuals except for homosexual relationships with adolescent boys.[7] It was considered unmanly for adult men to be sexually penetrated.[8] Homosexual prostitution or procurement was a crime. Assault or coercion of very young boys was unacceptable. Plato's proposed legal code accepted voluntary sex between an adult male and a younger man, but it proposed that a man be punished by death if he violated a free woman or a boy.[9] By addressing both heterosexual and homosexual relations, the *Oath* acknowledges the different cultural norms that applied to these actions as it asserted that both were unacceptable during the medical encounter.

. . . BOTH OF THE FREE AND OF THE SLAVES

The *Oath* explicitly disavowed sexual relations with slaves. This statement makes little sense to the modern ear. Slavery is immoral; we cannot define an injustice against a class of persons in a way that implicitly accepts the intrinsic immorality of the class itself. A third of the people in Greece were slaves.[10] The moral tensions with Athenian ideals were recognized, and Athens at one point even passed an abolition law that was revoked on a technicality.[11] Most slaves were aliens captured in war; thus they were stigmatized three times, as barbarians,[12] as enemies,[13] and as slaves. In the play *Hecabe*, Euripides gives voice to such persons in a speech by the conquered princess, Polyxena:

> Now, I am a slave. That name alone, being new to me makes me in love with death. Then, chance might give me a harsh-minded master who, having paid money for me, would send me to his kitchen—sister of Hector and many other royally born—to make bread, sweep the house, stand weaving at the loom: day after day of bitterness! And, some bought slave would claim my bed, soiling what kings once sued to have.[14]

Slaves were subject to forced servitude as concubines and were also worked as prostitutes. Aristophanes, a playwright, describes the sexual vulnerability of slave women through a man's speech:

> So now I can turn to the pleasures I'd always have chosen if I could, like finding my neighbor's young slave-girl in the act of purloining some wood, and grab-

bing her tight (for never have I known her to say "I will not"). And lifting her up to amuse her, then having it off on the spot.[15]

In this culture, a disavowal of paid, forced, or consensual sexual acts with slaves was not a given. Medical case records describe owners' bringing slave prostitutes to physicians for treatment. It should be noted, however, that notwithstanding the disavowal of sexual relations with slaves during the course of a clinical visit, it appears that physicians treated slaves differently than free people.[16]

One can speculate about two reasons why the *Oath* specifically condemned sexual relations with slaves during clinical visits. Perhaps it was a practical ethic; to wit: "The profession's reputation is harmed when people see a physician exploiting his privileges or power for personal sexual gratification." This possibility is suggested by this passage from the ancient Greek medical work called *Physician*:

> In every social relation, he [the physician] will be fair, for fairness is of great service. The intimacy also between physician and patient is close. Patients in fact put themselves into the hands of their physician and at every moment he meets women, maidens and possessions very precious indeed. So towards all these self-control must be used.[17]

Alternatively, perhaps it reflected a nascent view of social justice within Greek society that empathized with the degraded state of slavery, as suggested by the humanistic portrayals of slaves in Greek drama and the debate about abolition. These two views are not incompatible with each other.

HYBRIS

The greater significance of the words on sexual relations may lie in how they may shed light on the meaning of "voluntary and destructive injustice." The *Oath* posits sexual acts in the house of the ill as an example of a "voluntary and destructive injustice" and thus potentially clarifies a sense of the meaning of that larger class. That larger class could well be the set of injustices that were known as *hubris* or *hybris*.

Hybris was a self-indulgent vaunting or exploitation of one's power in order to dominate or dishonor.[18] In its most common usage, it differed from the modern dramaturgical concept of impious pride that is seen as the central character flaw driving such tragedies as *Oedipus Rex*. A modern synonym might be "arrogance that dishonors," in which case this passage from the *Oath* would read: "while refraining from destructive acts of arrogance that dishonor. . . ." The opposite of this important and legally punishable injustice was to being sensible, careful, disciplined, moral, or chaste rather than being "submissive" or "wimpy." Hybris was an injustice against the community, not just the individual victim, and thus it was a crime whose penalties could be as severe as death. Civil suits could recover monetary damages or other forms of satisfaction.[19]

There are several reasons why it seems fair to conclude that physicians would think about "voluntary and destructive injustice" as a form of hybris. First, it was a civil as well as criminal offense and thus extended beyond what was required by law. Second, hybris presumed an advantage in terms of status, opportunity, or power that a physician as a respected guest who was granted great intimacy would be well placed to abusively exploit. Third, it included actions that could be physically violent, or verbal or nonverbal insults to honor.[20] Athens explicitly applied hybris to instances of sexual abuse, exploitation, and assault (especially of children). In such usage it included acts that were either coercive or consensual and ranged from rape to seduction. Fourth, many Greek writers analogized a just society to a healthy body.[21] In that metaphor, hybris was seen as akin to an imbalance of humors—a fascinating link between health and ethics that would have plausibly been appealing to physicians. One might object that if the *Oath* meant to refer to hybris, then it would have used the word. The *Oath's* authors, however, proceeded from the principles of benefit and justice to specific examples without using intermediate ethical terms.[22] Though hybris was a transitional category that encompassed an important and diverse group of injustices, it was also the subject of a great deal of technical legal debate. It is not surprising that the *Oath* steered clear of this somewhat messy intermediate moral category.

Along with hybris, it must be noted that the *Oath* also does not use another term that is often cited as the paramount principle of Hippocratic medical ethics: "First, do no harm." Neither the *Oath* nor any Greek medical treatise contains such a phrase. The closest likeness is in *Epidemics I*: "Practice two things in your dealings with disease: either help or do not harm the patient."[23] Jonsen notes that Galen rephrased that passage by adding "above all" before the injunction to benefit the patient. Jonsen translates Galen's modification as follows: "The physician must aim above all at helping the sick; if he cannot, he should not harm them."[24] No one knows how or when "First, do no harm" came to be attributed to Hippocratic medicine or how it ascended to such mythic primacy.

Traces of the history of "do no harm" are known. In 416 BCE, about the time when the *Oath* was written, Nicias, an Athenian general and politician, spoke against what he accurately judged would be a disastrous military expedition to Sicily. He called upon the chair of the Athenian Council to "be the physician of your misguided city . . . the virtue of men in office is briefly this, to do their country as much good as they can, or in any case no harm that they can avoid."[25] An 1845 medical ethics book says: "No physician should ever forget the unbending moral precept: do not harm."[26] In 1863, Florence Nightingale wrote a popular work on hospital architecture that included the remark: "It may seem a strange principle to enunciate as the very first requirement in a hospital that it should do the sick no harm".[27] "First, do no harm" has a dubious provenance and is of overrated utility.

All therapies entail risks. A physician could not perform any surgery or administer any drug (even one dose of penicillin that could cause a lethal allergic reaction) if he or she was obliged to avoid the chance of harm. The pursuit of therapy—any therapy—represents a decision that the probability and magnitude of benefits outweigh the chance and severity of harms. This clinical calculation accepts risks rather than avoiding them. The Greek advice to "Practice two things in your dealings with disease: either help or do not harm the patient," implicitly admits the possibility of undertaking risky therapies while endeavoring to reduce those risks. It is worthier of Hippocratic Medicine than "Do no harm."

           *   *   *

VOLUNTARY AND DESTRUCTIVE INJUSTICE IN MEDICINE TODAY

If this chapter followed the precedent of previous chapters, it would now recount a case in which a physician abused a patient's trust. I have heard of, or read about, physicians who have sexually or financially exploited patients.[28] Research suggests that from two to nine percent of physicians have had a sexual contact with a patient.[29] There is even a book about physicians who were serial killers.[30] I have never met such a physician or sat in judgment of one, however. I have never treated a patient who has been harmed in such a way. The overwhelming majority of physicians are decent people who work ethically at their demanding careers.

It is more instructive to consider a voluntary and destructive injustice that is paradoxically both more important and more subtle. A substantial body of research consistently shows that physicians in the United States do not respond equally to indications for treatment in persons who are African American, American Indian, or Hispanic.[31] Physicians tend to underestimate the pain and administer insufficient amounts of pain-killing medicine to minority patients diagnosed with cancer or who have broken major bones in their bodies.[32] Similar patterns of under-treatment are seen for persons of color who present with heart attacks,[33] the warning signs of stroke,[34] colon cancer,[35] HIV-AIDS, diabetes, mental illness, and many other conditions. Such discrepancies do not disappear when researchers adjust the results for the patient's insurance status, wealth, or distance from medical treatment. People of color are also less likely to report that white physicians engage them in a participatory or interactional dialogue.[36]

This compelling evidence that the clinical decisions of well-meaning, experienced physicians are shaped by social bias obliges each physician to critically examine his or her own practice. That kind of moral vigilance is obliged by the vow to guard one's integrity in a pure and holy way. Yet this vow to keep "far from all voluntary and destructive injustice" takes us further. Given that research has found an unjust and harmful racial pattern of clinical decisions, a physician who arrogantly dismisses the personal challenge posed by that research risks committing a hybristic abuse of patients.

NOTES

1. Campbell ML. The Oath: An investigation of the injunction prohibiting physician–patient sexual relations. Perspect Biol Med 1989;32:300–8.

2. Dover 27, 34–6; Cohen (1991) 171–202.

3. Pomeroy (1975) 86-7, and Cohen (1991) 98–132.

4. Cohen (1991) 80, 178–83. A similar point applies to the confidentiality passage discussed in Chapter 12.

5. In addition to this account by Ctesias, there is the suspect story of Hagnodké that is attributed to Hyginus, a first-century BCE Roman scholar, who said the event occurred in 300 BCE (Fabula 274, 10–3). Hagnodké was reportedly an Athenian woman whose name meant "Chaste in Justice." She cut her hair short and learned medicine and midwifery. She practiced in Athens on a female clientele to whom she

revealed her true sex. Her patients were reluctant to see male doctors. Physicians had her prosecuted on a charge of sexual misconduct and corrupting men's wives. In court, she is said to have lifted up her cloak to reveal her sex. She was condemned to die for being a woman physician and practicing under false pretences. Athenian women successfully protested, Hagnodké was allowed to continue practicing medicine, and the law was amended so that freeborn Athenian women could be physicians for women patients. This story is widely reported in secondhand sources: Blundell (1985) 145; Bland (1994) 68, n98; Alic M (1986) 28–30; and Finnegan R. The Professional Careers: Women Pioneers and the Male Image Seduction. Classics Ireland, University College Dublin, Ireland 1995;2. Lloyd doubts the story because of a lack of confirming evidence of this case, of any law forbidding women to practice medicine, or of capital punishment for this kind of infraction Lloyd (1983) 70, n. 47.

6. Ctesias 41–2, trans. (from French) by Steven Miles.

7. Cantarella 17–53.

8. Halperin DM. "Why is Diotim a woman? Platonic eros and the figuration of gender," in Halperin, Winkerl, Zeitlin 258–308.

9. Plato. *Laws* 874 bc.

10. Hall in *Euripides* (1999) xxix.

11. Patterson 47–180 lucidly describes the institution of slavery and the moral and political debate about it in Greece's classic era.

12. The *Oath* is silent on injustice toward free aliens, and there are few clinical records describing the treatment of free aliens, who comprised one-twelfth of the Greek population. (Kudlien D. Medical ethics and popular ethics in Greece and Rome. Clio Med 1970;5:91–121.)

13. Aeschylus wrote two plays, *The Persians* and *The Suppliant Maidens*, that speak of the humanity of enemies of Athens and of the moral obligations to persons seeking asylum. Letters from the first century CE purport to describe a fifth century BCE request by a Persian ruler, who was hostile to the Greeks, for the services of a Greek physician (allegedly Hippocrates) to aid his state in dealing with an epidemic. The letters discuss the ethics of physicians coming to the aid of an enemy state. Letters 1–9, in Smith (1990). Jouanna also says that the letters are of late authorship, around the first century CE, but accepts the plausibility of the described event (Jouanna 20–2). Smith ([1970] 220) takes a skeptical view of the account—regarding this as late propaganda from Cos but is open to the reality of the central moral debate.

14. Euripides. *Hecabe* 359–6. Despite this degraded state, there was not an unlimited license to abuse slaves. For example, in Euripides' play *Andromache*, King Meneleus threatens to murder the slave woman Andromache. "Haven't I a right to my things?" he asks. Peleus rebukes him: "To care for, not to abuse. And not to slaughter." (Euripides. *Andromache* 585–6).

15. Aristophanes. *The Acharnians* p. 61.

16. Slaves are underrepresented in the medical treatises. They comprise only ten persent of the patients in the oldest case series (*Epidemics I* and *III*) and even fewer in the other case series *Epidemics V* and *VII*, whose authors appear to have served as trauma surgeons with armies as well as general public practice: they describe only five percent of their patients as slaves. There are accounts of treating slaves, e.g., *Epidemics* 4:38, 51, *Epidemics* 5:41. A typical account in *Epidemics V* goes: "The slave woman: after a potion she evacuated a little bile above, and choked; passed much below. She died that night. She was a barbarian" (*Epidemics* 5:35). It is not safe to assume that the treatment records accurately reflect the proportions of slave and free of those who were actually treated or received medical care. Even if slaves were under represented in the accounts of patients treated by Greek physicians, it would be unfair to simplistically blame materialistic or xenophobic physicians. Slave owners decided if and when a physician would be called to treat a slave. These owners had recourse to other kinds of healers, including healers who were slaves (*Epidemics 5:35*), medicines purchased in the market on the advice of a pharmacist, and temple healers. Such healers left scant records of their work. Plato notes that physicians who were slaves treated slaves by prescribing treatment but that they were not bound to give comparable education or obtain consent (*Laws 4.720a–d*). Greek physicians did note differences with regard to the epidemiology of disease in slaves and freemen (Jouanna 116).

17. *Physician I.*

18. Cantarella 43; Cohen (1991) 98–132, 178–183; Cohen (1995) 87–162; and MacDowell DM. Hybris in Athens, Greece and Rome 1976;23:14–31.

19. Cohen 83–88, 218–40.

20. Cohen (1995) 147–9.

21. Hurwitz MS. "Justice and the Metaphor of Medicine in Early Greek Thought," in Irani and Silver, 69–73.

22. It went directly from benefit and justice to the examples of deadly drugs and abortive pessaries, and from benefit and injustice to the examples of sexual acts and revealing secrets.

23. *Epidemics* I:XI. The commonly cited Jones translation follows Littré and goes: "As to diseases, make a habit of two things—to help, or *at least* do no harm" (Hippocrates [1923a]). Jonsen notes that the Greek text does not contain the words "at least." Jonsen AR. "Do No Harm." Ann Int Med 1978;88:827–32. I have used a later translation (Hippocrates [1950]).

24. Jonsen, op. cit., quoting Galen. *Commentarium I in Hippocratis libri I Epidemiorum c. 50*. Leipzig, C Cnoblochius, 1828, vol. 17A, p. 148.

25. *Thucydides* 6.14

26. Jonsen (op. cit.) quoting Simon M. Deontologie medicale. Paris: JB Baillière, 1845, p. 269.

27. Nightingale ix.

28. Garfinkel PE, Dorian B, Sadavoy J, Bagby RM. Boundary violations and departments of psychiatry. Can J Psychiatry 1997;42:764-70. Anonymous. Sexual misconduct in the practice of medicine. Council on Ethical and Judicial Affairs, American Medical Association. JAMA 1991;266:2741-5.

29. Gartrell NK, Milliken N, Goodson WH III, et al. Physician–patient sexual contact. Prevalence and problems. West J Med 1992;157:139-43.

30. Iserson.

31. Committee on Understanding and Eliminating Racial and Ethnic Disparities in Health Care.

32. Anderson KO, Mendoza TR, Valero V et al. Minority cancer patients and their providers: pain management attitudes and practice. Cancer 2000;88:1929-38. Todd KH, Samaroo N, Hoffman JR. Ethnicity as a risk factor for inadequate emergency department analgesia. JAMA 1993;269:1537-9. Todd KH, Deaton C, D'Adamo AP, Goe L. Ethnicity and analgesic practice. Ann Emerg Med 2000;35:11-6.

33. Peterson ED, Wright SM, Daley J, Thibault GE. Racial variation in cardiac procedure use and survival following acute myocardial infarction in the Department of Veterans Affairs. JAMA 1994;271:1175-80.

34. Mitchell JB, Ballard DJ, Matchar DB, et al. Racial variation in treatment for transient ischemic attacks: Impact of participation by neurologists. Health Serv Res 2000;34:1413-28.

35. Ball JK, Elixhauser A. Treatment differences between blacks and whites with colorectal cancer. Med Care 1996;34:970-84.

36. Cooper-Patrick L, Gallo JJ, Gonzales JJ et al. Race, gender, and partnership in the patient–physician relationship. JAMA 1999;282:583-9.

12

DISCRETION IN SPEECH

AND ABOUT WHATEVER I MAY SEE OR HEAR IN TREATMENT, OR
EVEN WITHOUT TREATMENT, IN THE LIFE OF HUMAN BEINGS,
THINGS THAT SHOULD NOT EVER BE BLURTED OUT OUTSIDE, I
WILL REMAIN SILENT, HOLDING SUCH THINGS TO BE *ARRĒTA*
[UNUTTERABLE, SACRED, NOT TO BE DIVULGED].

This passage is usually read as a promise to respect the confidentiality of information that a patient has disclosed and information about that person's medical conditions. Arras says that this clinical principle has a utilitarian origin, arising from the insight that patients will not disclose necessary information unless clinicians promise confidentiality.[1] Carrick asserts that this passage is a disavowal of physicians' using privileged information for personal gain, though its wording seems to say that disclosure itself, rather than the *use* of the disclosed information, is the transgression.[2] Kudlien says that this passage forbids disclosing state secrets.[3] Though Greek oaths cementing political alliances often swore secrecy in affairs of state, this seems an unlikely meaning for a physician's oath. As with other passages of the *Oath*, one must look to the cultural context and differences with modern medical ethics to try to discern its meaning.

Modern medical ethics distinguishes between *confidentiality* and *privacy*.

Confidentiality refers to safeguarding information. American courts have clarified a special sense of medical *privacy* through decisions regarding the right to obtain contraceptives and abortions and to refuse life-sustaining treatment. In this sense, *privacy* refers to the personal freedom to affirm particular values and to make important life choices based on them.[4] For example, in 1965, the United States Supreme Court overturned state laws that prohibited married couples from obtaining contraceptives and barred physicians from prescribing them. The Court recognized a married couple's right to privacy about whether and why to use contraceptives.[5] In everyday speech, *confidentiality* and *privacy* are often used interchangeably, or we say that "confidentiality requires privacy;" i.e., a room where the physician–patient discussion cannot be overheard. To avoid confusion, I shall use *seclusion* to refer to an unmonitored place for the clinical visit where having a confidential communication is possible. In any case, this passage refers to confidentiality and not to the contemporary medical ethics of the right to privacy.

It may be possible to trace our modern medical ethic of respect for the confidentiality of medical information to this passage, but we should be cautious in doing so. Our idea of confidential medical care did not exist in ancient Greece. Greece did not seclude clinical care as we do today. Physicians took histories, examined patients, gave prognoses, and practiced surgery in public or in houses as relatives and strangers looked on.[6] Male guardians or owners were entitled to medical information about women, children, and slaves, and they were empowered to dictate medical choices as well. The medical treatises published the names, addresses, and intimate details of many patients:

In Larissa, the menses of Gorgia's wife had stopped. . . . [7]
In Abdera, Nicodemus after venery and drunkenness was seized with fever.[8]
Chaerion who lay at the house of Delias took a fever as a result of drinking.[9]
Timochares in winter had catarrhs. When he had sexual activity, all was dried up.[10]
In Larissa, the servant [slave?] of Dyseris when she was young whenever she had sexual intercourse suffered much pain but otherwise was without distress.[11]
Nicippus had a wet dream in fever and it made him no worse. The same thing repeatedly occurred and did not harm him. It was predicted that it would end when the fever reached crisis, and so it did. Critias was upset by dreams that cause erections.[12]

It is not clear how these names came to be recorded, but there is no reason to believe that they are pseudonyms. At the time they were written, Asclepian temples were inscribed with testimonials giving the names, diseases, methods of divination, and clinical outcomes attesting to the successful treatment of the ill supplicants.[13] If Greek physicians' medical records are modeled after these temple testimonials, they used real names. Greek medical treatises asserted that location, ethnicity, and occupation were epidemiologically important. It is reasonable to believe that addresses, jobs, and habits were details to be accurately noted by practitioners of the observational science of medicine. Apparently, either the information given in the medical treatises was not covered by the *Oath* or this passage refers to other kinds of information.

The *Oath's* promise to respect confidentiality refers to a particular set of information: "Of whatever I see . . . *that should not be aired*, I will remain silent." One clue about the nature of this information is that breaches of confidentiality seem to be the second example of how a physician should refrain "from all voluntary and destructive injustice." If so, such transgressions would be a hubristic abuse of the ethic of hospitality, *xenos*, as discussed in the previous chapter. If this reading is correct, then this passage refers to a physician who used privileged information to dishonor persons. Greeks did not see words as simply conveying information: words were powerful things that charmed and polluted as well.[14]

Further support for the view that this passage disavows dishonoring patients is found in its use of *arrēta* as the moral principle by which transgression of disclosure is be morally evaluated. Jones and von Staden translate *arrēta* as "holy secrets" or "unutterable [sacred, not to be divulged]."[15] It is also defined as "profane things" or "deeds too shameful to be spoken of." *Arrēta* is not simply boorish talk or name-dropping; nor is it like our casual use of the word "profanity." The word *arrēta* is further clarified by its use in Greek plays of the *Oath's* time. In *Oedipus at Colonus*, Creon vilifies Oedipus as a, "father-killer, worse, a creature so corrupt, exposed as the mate, the unholy husband of his own mother."[16] Oedipus offers this rebuttal:

> OEDIPUS: Shameless—where do you think your insults do more damage, my old
> age or yours? . . . [My] mother, wretched man, have you no shame? Your own
> sister! Her marriage—forcing me to talk of that marriage. Oh, I'll tell it all, I

won't be silent, not now, you and your blasphemous mouth have gone too far. She was my mother, yes, she bore me . . . I knew nothing, she knew nothing. . . . But you slander her and me of your own free will. But you are not just; you are one who considers it a fine thing to utter every sort of word, both those which are sanctioned and those which are forbidden [*arrēta*].[17]

The medical treatises did not give examples of physicians saying "things that should not ever be blurted out outside," but it seems clear that this kind of profane speech, especially when disavowed by an oath, would have polluted or dishonored the physician as well as the person of whom the physician spoke. In that the physician revealed these things "outside," this passage speaks of the need for a moral coherence between a physician's personal and professional life.

That moral coherence was explicitly articulated in a preceding passage: "In a pure and holy way I will guard my life and my *techné*." The confidentiality passage closed the stanza that began with entering a person's private world with a rule for the physician who has returned to the public world with private information. The words "whatever I may see or hear in treatment, or even without treatment" recognized that people tell private things to physicians even outside of clinical encounters—for example, at social gatherings. The vow to refrain from speaking of patients in a profane manner covers any information about a patient (and probably the patient's household as well), no matter how or where it was obtained.

*   *   *

CASE 12.1 One night, I was in an intensive care unit waiting for confirmation that a therapy was helping a seriously ill patient. I was sitting beside the computer terminal that would deliver the lab data I needed. I idly entered my five-digit employee code to gain access to the health plan's database. I entered my own name in the field for a patient's name. Since I am not my own doctor, I had no special privilege to this medical data. The computer displayed my address, birthday, place of employment, and the name of my physician. I now had enough information to stalk myself or to forge an identity for commercial transactions. Icons, menus, and clicks of the mouse took me to screens displaying clinics I had visited, lab results, and prescriptions. My employer had an access code: did he know that I was on medicines for a psychiatric illness? I saw my partner's name and gender but refrained from looking up her medical record, though I could have. I saw that the health plan could have, but did not record my faith or whether I had a Living Will. I saw my eye clinic appointments. Any of the thousands of people with an access code could make a list for a laser surgery clinic that might like to do some targeted marketing of their services. I did not see any genetic tests that might interest a company selling nursing home insurance. Obviously, there were no data suggesting that I had had an abortion, though such data would have been accessible. Screen after screen—my life was bared to anyone with a five-digit code and access to any of thousands of data terminals.

People are deeply concerned about protecting the confidentiality of their medical information. They fear that they will not get health insurance if an insurer finds out that they have been sick. They are concerned that an employer will limit their work or promotions if certain medical conditions become known. They do not want to receive advertisements because a physician, clinic, or pharmacist has sold personal medical data to a company.[18] They are horrified when a drug company inadvertently broadcasts the names and e-mail addresses of people who are taking its antidepressants. Young people are more willing to seek help with contraceptives, sexually transmitted diseases, or drug abuse if they are assured of confidentiality.[19] A person may even fear disclosure of confidential information after his or her death and, except for a death certificate, medical information is confidential after death.[20] The promise of confidentiality is essential to an open communication within a trusting physician–patient relationship.

Confidentiality can be breached in many ways. Physicians or medical students talk with each other in hospital elevators.[21] A clinic clerk gossips in a small town. A person who opposes abortion photographs people entering a clinic. A drugstore sells customer names to a drug company that does a direct mailing to try to get a person to switch to their products. A medical record is mailed to a health insurer who could use data from a genetic test that was performed to help a patient to bar that person from obtaining disability or long-term-care insurance.[22] A database or e-mail between a patient and a physician is inadequately protected.[23] Notations about a person's sexual orientation, history of having an abortion, or psychiatric care may be noted and transcribed by another physician and then released to another party who has requested the second physician's record. Given the diversity of ways that information is shared and accessible, it is not surprising that physicians are uncertain about how to honor their duty to protect the confidentiality of medical information or to advise the patient of the long-term consequences of any notation in a medical record.[24]

Medical ethics standards are difficult to devise because perfect confidentiality is not possible, desirable, or a reasonable right to affirm. Employers and insurers claim that patients "voluntarily" waive confidentiality so that the provision and payment of care can be monitored to keep costs lower.[25] Large electronic databases of health-care encounters from which identifying data have been largely stripped are necessary for research to improve public health.[26] Public health officials should know when the death rate of babies at a specific hospital is too high so the problem can be[27] addressed. An unconscious patient with a medical emergency can be saved if a physician can get medical information from another physician about an underlying disease or allergy to a drug.[28] Clinicians must report their suspicions that a child or vulnerable older person has been abused, neglected, or exploited in order to protect the vulnerable.[29] A psychiatrist may have a duty to break confidence if she learns that a patient plans to harm another specific person.[30] Physicians who are impaired by alcoholism must agree to be monitored during rehabilitation.[31] Some states have tried to require physicians to report illegal immigrants who come for health care, even though such reporting may result in a fear of seeking health care, or delayed treatment for infectious or lethal diseases. Though a minor often has a legal and moral right to receive confidential care, protecting that confidentiality is difficult when it comes to seeking reimbursement through family health insurance.[32]

Accordingly, the rules and ethics of confidentiality are complex. Policies to define the access and safeguarding of data are a top concern.[33] The policies, ethics, and laws pertaining to confidentiality are rapidly evolving, and each physician honors this commitment by keeping abreast of those developments and implements them in the spirit of protecting the patient's interests.

✻   ✻   ✻

CASE 12.2 Maria was a prisoner who was admitted to a hospital with a bleeding stomach ulcer. The clinical goal was to treat her bleeding and send her back to prison where she would die from her advanced AIDS within the next month or two. Her weight had fallen to less than a hundred pounds and she was too weak to lift herself from the bed. She begged me to send her to a nursing home so that she could die near her mother's home. I asked the resident physician to arrange it.

He reacted negatively, "She was sentenced to prison; she should stay there. You do not even know her crime. It is not our job to get involved in this."

I acknowledged that her punishment was the state's responsibility but also noted that our duty, as her physician, would be to support her request to be with her mother as she died. We arranged with the Department of Corrections to transfer her to the custody of a nursing home where she died with her mother at her side a few weeks later.

The Oath offers a second way to the ethics of things a physician may not speak of. In using *arrēta* to define the information that should not be spoken of outside, the *Oath* may not have been speaking of the modern preoccupation with confidential medical information. Rather, it may have been a disavowal of the voluntary and destructive injustice of speaking about patients in a dishonoring way. In this sense, it would be profane to speak of Maria's prison crime or prison sentence as being any more relevant to a physician's advocacy for a home death with her mother at her side than the crime or sentence would be relevant to the decision to treat her bleeding ulcer with a blood transfusion. Even Oedipus merited a home to die in. By the same token, Shem's notorious book *The House of God*, in which physicians hybristically speak of patients as junkies, gomers, dirtballs, drunks, bounces, hits, or vegetables, is also a litany of words that "should not ever be blurted out outside" by a person who has sworn to be a physician.[34]

NOTES

1. Arras JD. A method in search of a purpose: The internal morality of medicine. J Med Phil 2001;6:643–62. Arras is not specifically analyzing this passage of the *Oath* but is looking at this duty as being intrinsically necessary for medicine.
2. Carrick 93. Carrick's proposal that focuses the scope of this passage to physicians who exploit private information for personal gain does not give full weight to the ethics of shame and dishonor in Greece as is discussed later in this chapter.
3. Kudlien F. Medical ethics and popular ethics in Greece and Rome. Clio Med 1970;5:91–121 at 110.
4. Faden and Beachamp 39–41.
5. *Griswold vs. Connecticut*, 381 U.S. 479 (1965)
6. Jouanna 75.
7. *Epidemics 5:11*.
8. *Epidemics III: (sixteen Cases): X.*
9. *Epidemics III; Case V.*
10. *Epidemics 5:72.*
11. *Epidemics V:25.*

12. *Epidemics* 4:57.

13. Aleshire.

14. Entralgo PL (1970, 32–171.) This power of words is how curses could cause disease that could be cured by the supplications of Asclepiad healers. This power also explains Greek concern about public impiety as damaging the world.

15. Jones (Hippocrates [1923]). von Staden H. "In a pure and holy way": Personal and professional conduct in the Hippocratic Oath. J Hist Med Allied Sci 1966;51:406–8.

16. Sophocles. *Oedipus at Colonus* 1076–8.

17. Sophocles. *Oedipus at Colonus* 1095–1105, 1117–26, 1143–46.

18. Lo B, Alpers A. Uses and abuses of prescription drug information in pharmacy benefits management programs. JAMA 2000;283:801–6. Anonymous. Statement of principles: The sale and use of data on individual physicians' prescribing. Canadian Medical Association. CMAJ 1997;156:424A–D.

19. Ford CA, Millstein SG, Halpern-Felsher BL, Irwin CE Jr. Influence of physician confidentiality assurances on adolescents' willingness to disclose information and seek future health care. JAMA 1997;278:1029–34. Thrall JS, McCloskey L, Ettner SL, et al. Confidentiality and adolescents' use of providers for health information and for pelvic examinations. Arch Pediatr Adolresc Med 2000;154:885–92.

20. Maixner AH, Morin K. The Council on Ethical and Judicial Affairs, American Medical Association. Confidentiality of health information postmortem. Arch Pathol Lab Med 2001;125:1189–92

21. Ubel PA, Zell MM, Miller DJ, et al. Elevator talk: Observational study of inappropriate comments in a public space. Am J Med 1995;99:190–4.

22. Troy ES. The Genetic Privacy Act: An analysis of privacy and research concerns. Am J Law Med 1997;25:256–72, 230. Cunningham GC. The genetics revolution: Ethical, legal, and insurance concerns. Postgrad Med 2000;108:193–6. Kulynych J, Korn D. Use and disclosure of health information in genetic research: Weighing the impact of the new federal medical privacy rule. Am J Law Med 2002; 28:309–24.

23. Mandl KD, Kohane IS, Brandt AM. Electronic patient–physician communication: Problems and promise. Ann Intern Med 1998;129:495–500. Miller RA, Schaffner KF, Meisel A. Ethical and legal issues related to the use of computer programs in clinical medicine. Ann Intern Med 1985;102:529–37.

24. Shrier I, Green S, Solin J, et al. Knowledge of and attitude toward patient confidentiality within three family medicine teaching units. Acad Med 1998;73:710–2.

25. Rischitelli DG. The confidentiality of medical information in the workplace. J Occup Environ Med 1995;37:583–93. McCunney RJ. Preserving confidentiality in occupational medical practice. Am Fam Physician 1996;53:1751–60.

26. Korn D. Medical information privacy and the conduct of biomedical research. Acad Med 2000;75:963–8. Simon GE, Unutzer J, Young BE, Pincus HA. Large medical databases, population-based research, and patient confidentiality Am J Psychiatr 2000;157:1731–7.

27. Geltman PL. Meyers AF. Immigration reporting laws: ethical dilemmas in pediatric practice. Am J Pub Health 1998;88:967–8.

28. Larkin GL, Moskop J, Sanders A, Derse A. The emergency physician and patient confidentiality: A review. Ann Emerg Med 1994;24:1161–7.

29. Guidelines for managing domestic abuse when male and female partners are patients of the same physician. The Delphi Panel and the Consulting Group. JAMA 1997;278:851–7. Halverson KC, Elliott BA, Rubin MS, Chadwick DL. Legal considerations in cases of child abuse. Primary Care; Clinics in Office Practice 1993;20:407–16. Hazzard WR. Elder abuse: Definitions and implications for medical education. Acad Med 1995;70:979–81.

30. Felthous AR. The clinician's duty to protect third parties. Psychiatr Clin North Am 1999;22:49–60.

31. American Psychiatric Association. Position statement on confidentiality of medical records: Does the physician have a right to privacy concerning his or her own medical records? Am J Psychiatry 1984;141:331–2.

32. Anonymous. The adolescent's right to confidential care when considering abortion. American Academy of Pediatrics—Committee on Adolescence. Pediatr 1996;97:746–51. Weddle M, Kokotailo P. Adolescent substance abuse: Confidentiality and consent. Pediatr Clin North Am 2002;49:301–15. Chilton L, Berger JE, Melinkovich P, et al. American Academy of Pediatrics' Pediatric Practice Action Group and Task Force on Medical Informatics. Privacy protection and health information: Patient rights and pediatrician responsibilities. Pediatrics 1999;104:973–7

33. Dodek DY, Dodek A. From Hippocrates to facsimile. Protecting patient confidentiality is more difficult and more important than ever before. CMAJ 1997; 156:847–52.

34. Shem.

III

IN WHAT WAY ARE PHYSICIANS ACCOUNTABLE?

IF I RENDER THIS OATH FULFILLED, AND IF I DO NOT BLUR AND
CONFOUND IT [MAKING IT TO NO EFFECT] MAY IT BE
[GRANTED] TO ME TO ENJOY THE BENEFITS BOTH OF LIFE AND
OF *TECHNÉ*, BEING HELD IN GOOD REPUTE AMONG ALL HUMAN
BEINGS FOR TIME ETERNAL. IF, HOWEVER, I TRANSGRESS AND
PERJURE MYSELF, THE OPPOSITE OF THESE.

The *Oath's* two closing sentences are so tightly intertwined that they may be
considered as a single passage. On a quick reading, this closing seems simply to be a final attestation of sincerity. On closer inspection, it speaks of two
moral issues. First, it defines several distinct ways by which a physician is to
understand how these vows are binding. The physician must not be committing perjury, must not blur and confound the words, and must not transgress
against the vows proper. Second, the physician swears to stand under the
judgment of "all human beings for time eternal." In that swearing an oath
was voluntary, a modern reader might question the importance of the act of
making an oath. In ancient Greece, an oath set the swearer apart from the
ordinary moral obligations.

Ancient Greece's system of laws coexisted with communal moral traditions.
Though oaths were legally enforceable, they went beyond the law. They were
a means by which a person voluntarily assumed duties beyond those that were

legally required. The community morally evaluated a person who had sworn an oath according to how well those exceptional duties were honored rather than according to the standards that applied to ordinary people. In this way, an oath brought exceptional honor or disrepute. This passage from the *Oath* is worth scrutinizing because it describes how a physician is bound to the antecedent vows and describes who evaluates how well the physician lived up to those commitments. In short, this closing defines the power of the *Oath* to set the terms for assessing the trustworthiness of the physician.

13

A TRUSTWORTHY PROFESSION

IF I RENDER THIS OATH FULFILLED, AND IF I DO NOT BLUR AND
CONFOUND IT [MAKING IT TO NO EFFECT] MAY IT BE
[GRANTED] TO ME TO ENJOY THE BENEFITS BOTH OF LIFE AND
OF *TECHNÉ* (ART AND SCIENCE), BEING HELD IN GOOD REPUTE
AMONG ALL HUMAN BEINGS FOR TIME ETERNAL. IF, HOWEVER, I
TRANSGRESS AND PERJURE MYSELF, THE OPPOSITE OF THESE.

WHAT IS AN OATH?

Oaths bind promises. The *Oath* simply puts the swearer's character on the line
for human judgment on whether the physician has honored the pledges to learn,
to teach, to sustain the development of medicine, to benefit the ill, and to shun
injustice. It is not a legal code. It is not a holy scripture. It is neither a prayer
for healing powers nor an affirmative answer to a divine call to be a doctor. It
is not a contract with a god that says: "If God grants me healing powers, I will
do this."

The playwright Euripides has Medea, who is about to murder her own children and her husband's new wife, define the difference between a promise and
an oath as she negotiates for the sanctuary she will need after committing the
crime. Without revealing her homicidal plan, she asks her friend Aegeus to
grant her refuge when she leaves her home. After he says that he will offer her

a home, she asks him to swear an oath to that effect. The following conversation ensues:

> MEDEA: Now, confirm your promise with an oath and all is well between us.
> AEGEUS: Why? Do you not trust me?
> MEDEA: I trust you; but I have enemies . . . once you are bound by an oath you will not give me up. . . . But if your promise is verbal, and not sworn to the gods, perhaps you will make friends with them and agree to do what they demand. I've no power on my side while they have wealth and all the resources of a royal house.
> AEGEUS: Your forethought is remarkable; but since you wish it, I've no objection. In fact, the taking of an oath safeguards me; since I can confront your enemies with a clear excuse while you have full security. So, name your gods.[1]

Aegeus unwittingly swears to protect the perpetrator of a savage deed. Like other oaths described in Greek drama and history, his oath binds his promise, but there is no assurance that the sworn deed will be good or evil, prudent or rash.

Oaths have been called the "connective tissue" of ancient Greece.[2] They sealed political allegiances and united cults, guilds, and brotherhoods. They bound citizens of an endangered city-state when expediency might counsel flight or betrayal. In one medical analogy, this use of an oath might bind a physician to serve a community despite the personal danger posed by an infectious epidemic of disease.[3] Persons swearing oaths to each other often took the same gods and laws and even established kinship obligations to each other. For example, the physician pledges to regard a teacher as a parent and to care for a teacher in the event of his infirmity. Oaths implied long-term duties, and the individual also assumed responsibility for the far-reaching consequences of honoring or breaking this commitment. These words imputed to Apollo's Oracle by the historian Herodotus described the effects of breaking an oath to Glaucus, who had asked if he might violate an oath:

> Today, indeed Glaucus, son of Epicydes, it is more profitable to prevail by false swearing and rob them of their money. Swear if you will; for death awaits even the true-swearer. Yet an oath has a son, nameless, without hands or feet, but swift to pursue until he has seized and destroys utterly the race and house of the perjured one. The children of him who keeps his oath are happier hereafter.[4]

As an injustice, it weakened the fabric of the world and society.

When oaths were sufficiently devalued, a society could fall. Thucydides offers this view of the effects of the devaluing of oaths on the negotiations to end the ruinous Peloponnesian wars:

> Oaths of reconciliation, being offered on either side to meet an immediate difficulty, only held good so long as no other weapon was at hand. . . . Thus, religion was in honor with neither party; but the use of fair phrases to arrive at guilty ends was in high reputation. . . . The ancient simplicity in which honor so largely entered was laughed down and disappeared; and society became divided into camps in which no man trusted his fellow. To put an end to this, there was neither promise to be depended upon, nor oath that could command respect; but all parties dwelling rather in their calculation upon the hopelessness of a permanent state of things, were more intent upon self-defense than capable of confidence. In this contest, the blunter were more successful. . . . In the confusion into which life was now thrown in the cities, human nature, always rebelling against the law and now its master, gladly showed itself ungoverned in passion, above respect for justice. . . .[5]

From this perspective, oaths are not simply personal promises; they are a social institution. Society rests on the integrity of individual oaths. So too, those who made and swore this oath would have seen physicians as a group being upheld by the trustworthiness with which each physician made and kept his commitment. The *Oath's* closing lines define the dimensions of the expected fidelity.

IF I DO NOT BLUR AND CONFOUND IT . . . OR TRANSGRESS AND PERJURE

Many commentators skip past these words as if they are merely repetitious signifiers of commitment to the specific promises stated in the body of the *Oath*. But the *Oath* has not used the rhetorical adornment of redundancy, and there is no reason to believe that it would have started to do so at this point. These words described four distinct ways that a physician promised to reflect on and keep his commitments. These standards were: perjury, transgression, blurring and confounding. Perjury and transgressing are the most clear cut. Falsely swearing an oath—perjury—had been regarded as immoral since at least the time of Homer. In Athens, lying under oath was a crime. Transgression refers to simple noncompliance with the vows. The *Oath* puts the physician under a broader obligation than to not swear falsely or subsequently break the vows. Physicians vowed to not "blur and confound" the terms of the *Oath*. "Blur" seems to have referred to employing wily rationalizations to obscure the *Oath's* meaning. Von Staden translates "confound" as making the *Oath* "without effect"[6] in which case "confound" may have referred to using technicalities to evade the *Oath's* intent. Phaedra, in a play by Euripides, spoke of the complexity of honestly keeping a vow. She was discussing temptations she faced to keep her marriage vow and of the kind of moral vigilance that is required to live a good life:

> Many a time in night's long empty spaces, I have pondered on the causes of a life's shipwreck. I think that our lives are worse than the mind's quality would warrant. There are many who know virtue. We know the good; we apprehend it clearly. But we can't bring it to achievement. Some are betrayed by their own laziness, and others value some other pleasure above virtue. . . . The proverb runs, "There is one thing alone that stands the brunt of life throughout its course, a quiet conscience," a just and quiet conscience whoever can attain it. . . . [The] deadly thing that devastates well-ordered cities and the homes of men—that's it, this art of over-subtle words.[7]

Phaedra's words pertain as well to oaths of medical ethics as they do to marriage vows. The *Oath* recognizes this difficulty where the physician vows to honor his commitments to the best of "my power and my judgment." Who judged whether physician lived up to his oath?

IN GOOD REPUTE AMONG ALL HUMAN BEINGS

It is remarkable that the *Oath* closed with a supplication to the judgment of the larger human community: "If I render this oath fulfilled . . . may it be granted to me to . . . [enjoy the benefits both of life and of *techné* (discussed in Chapter 8)] [and to be held] in good repute among all human beings." This entreaty seems to contradict those who see Hippocratic ethics as a convention for a morally insular guild.[8] Alternative possible closings illuminate the import of this phrase. If the ancient physicians saw themselves as an autonomous guild, the *Oath* might have ended, "I will accept the judgment and sanctions of eminent physicians as to whether I have honored these commitments." Alternatively, the *Oath* might have closed with an imprecation, "If I fulfill this oath, may the gods bless me; otherwise, may they curse me."[9] Greek physicians did not believe that sickness, healing, (or guilt[10]) was caused by divine curses and blessings. The closing appeal to the moral judgment of all human beings seems to invite a moral dialogue between the profession and the broader society.

This call for a moral dialogue between physicians and the larger human community also suggests a Greek position on what we now call the "internal morality of medicine." Advocates of that position believe that the experience of working as a physician confers an especially authoritative insight on what is required in the way of ethical behavior of a physician.[11] Others say that medical ethics is defined in the larger society. For example, modern respect for individualism has forged a doctrine of informed consent for the practice of medicine. A blended view sees medical ethics as the evolving outcome of an encounter between the moral traditions of medicine and changing social mores. In that blended view, the *Oath's* disavowal of sexual relations with patients endures, while its tacit acceptance of the propriety of a slave–physician relationship or a men-only profession is rightly rejected. In asking for a moral evaluation by the larger human community, the *Oath* seems to be open to something like a blended position in which society's time-tested moral views are the proper measure of the ethics of medicine. Of course, the blended position has a historical dimension. Good medical ethics is not defined by physicians' own traditions or authority but is continuously reevaluated by human cultural standards that were previously unknown and unenvisioned. Just as it does in evaluating a patient, the *Oath* explicitly asserts that observational time will refine an assessment of the condition, regimen, and prognosis of the body.

IN GOOD REPUTE . . . FOR TIME ETERNAL

In looking to a moral assessment of medicine by "all human beings for time eternal," the *Oath* made two additional points about medical ethics. First, it seems to have pointed to the potential of this medical ethics to change in light of evaluation by the future human community. This possibility should not be seen as evidence that the ancient Greeks believed the rules of ethics changed over time. Greeks were uncertain about human, moral, technological or political evolution.[12] It is more likely that this phrase suggests a willingness to

accept that the *understanding* of the ethics of medicine may become clearer
with further observation and reflection. In either case, the *Oath* does not seem
to have held itself out as a definitive statement of medical ethics. It offered its
conclusions as a human work to the human community.

Second, the *Oath's* invitation of moral evaluation by the future human community introduces a new mood: hopefulness. Until this point, its tone has been
solemn, even proud: "I will use regimens for the benefit of the ill." Though
the *Oath* expresses hope that a physician who honors these vows will be well
regarded, this optimism is tempered with a Greek tragic sense of history. This
is not surprising when one remembers that the *Oath* was written when Athens
was militarily defeated and financially ruined and the glory of the Parthenon
and Sophocles lay in the not so distant past. Other cultures were ascendant.
The Greeks saw that history did not necessarily reward virtue.[13] Good people
could be forgotten, remembered for a single misstep, or unjustly disparaged.
Though the *Oath* was sworn with enough confidence to invite disrepute or an
unhappy life on those who dishonored it, it appropriately closed on a note of
supplication: "may it be granted to me. . . ."

✳   ✳   ✳

CASE 13.1 I entered the Sarajevo hospital from a sidewalk carefully marked off
from hospital grounds that were studded with unexploded rocket grenades. Many
of windows had no glass. Mortars had opened patients' rooms to the air. A gap-
ing hole in a stairwell opened to a scenic view over the river toward the bluff the
shells had come from. The hospital was still treating patients.

It had trained Dr. Radovan Karadzic as a psychiatrist.[14] His former neighbors
sought treatment within its walls.

As president of the Bosnian Serb Republic, Dr. Karadzic oversaw the shell-
ing of Sarajevo and its hospital. He commanded snipers to fire on its citizens
and children as they tried to play, work, scavenge for food, and bury their dead.
He expelled more than 30,000 Muslims from a U.N. "safe area." He oversaw
the creation of rape centers and concentration camps where torture, starvation,
and summary executions were common.

I had taken my 17-year-old daughter with me as I performed a field evaluation for a group rebuilding the former Yugoslavia so that she could learn about
what I do and about what war is like. As we flew home, I asked her what she had
learned. She turned away from me and looked out the airplane window. After a
pause, she said, "My teachers told me that war is about trenches and torpedoes,
but that is only partly true. War is about men killing men and boys, and raping

and killing women and girls. It is bombed schools, bombed hospitals, bombed homes, and people who will be homeless forever."

CASE 13.2 In 1999, the Ministry of Justice of Turkey charged Dr. H. Zeki Uzun, a gynecologist in Turkey, with sedition. Dr. Uzun documented evidence of torture for the Human Rights Foundation of Turkey. He was arrested and his files were seized. He was kept in isolation, deprived of sleep, and interrogated. While imprisoned, he was beaten and kicked on the head and chest. A plastic bag was placed over his head to induce the feeling of suffocation. A bottle was inserted in his rectum, and his testicles were squeezed.

The *Oath* speaks of the judgment of history on physicians. We tend to think of the repute of physicians in smaller terms. We think of physicians who are sued for negligent care or for abandoning a patient in the middle of an operation so he can run to the bank and deposit a check. We think of the disrepute of physicians who are summoned before a Board of Medical Practice for sexually touching a patient. We think of the physicians who fraudulently bill insurance companies or Medicare for services. Apparently, ancient Greece did not envision malpractice suits, medical boards, and insurance oversight. Such forms of judging the reputation of physicians are hardly of the heroic scale of being assessed by "all human beings for time eternal." Greek virtue and honor had epic dimensions. Thus I believe that it is fair to close this examination of the *Oath's* last passage with a consideration of physicians and crimes against humanity.

In many countries, physicians assist with torture. They assist in ensuring that it causes pain without killing the prisoner. If the prisoner is not to be "disappeared," some physicians have helped devise methods including beatings, electric shock, suspension, cold hosing, near suffocation, threats, enacted executions, rape, and the torture of family members in front of the prisoner to minimize the physical evidence of torture. Some physicians falsely report that the person bears no sign of torture.[15] The United Nations' Convention Against Torture says that physicians should be educated about torture and its consequences so that victims can be properly treated and protected.[16] Torture is practiced in nearly half the countries of the world.

Humankind judges Dr. Karadzic and Dr. Uzun for their deeds as humans but also for the fact that they are physicians. Dr. Karadzic turned his medical ear away from those who were suffering when he could have aided them, and he misused his medical knowledge to enhance that suffering by devising, supervising, and implementing policies for starvation and psychological and physical torture.[17] An Interpol "Wanted Poster" lists the charges in the indictment: "Crimes against humanity, genocide, grave breaches of the 1949 Geneva Conventions, and violations of the law or customs of war."[18] There is a five-million-dollar award for his arrest. The World Medical Association has denounced him for not surrendering to the War Crimes Tribunal.[19]

By contrast, Dr. Uzun's honor seems enhanced, if such were possible, by virtue of his choice to forgo the comforts of a physician's life in order to uphold the commitments of the healing profession. Furthermore, the Turkish Medical Association, which has a distinguished history of resisting torture, sustained him through his trial and acquittal of all charges. He was also sustained by physicians in other countries, including the American College of Physicians, Physicians for Human Rights, the British Medical Association, and the Health Professionals Network of Amnesty International.[20] Dr. Uzun explains his ongoing commitment with these words: "I have been loyal to the Hippocratic Oath . . . and I will continue to perform my profession."[21]

Why was Dr. Uzun acquitted? Certainly, he was innocent of the charges. Justice, however, is hardly certain in countries where torture is practiced. At least one Turkish court has acknowledged that the *Oath* legitimizes work against torture by physicians. It pleases me to imagine that it has something to do with the moral sensibility of judges from a country that holds the ruins of Troy, where Podalirius, a son of Asclepius, began his travels down the coast to point his descendents' sails for the nearby island of Cos, the birthplace of Hippocrates.

NOTES

1. Euripides. *Medea* 729–46. See a similar account in *Iphigenia Among the Taurians* 745–53, in Morwood (1999).

2. A technical discussion of this can be found in Parker 186–7. Many accounts of how ancient Greek oaths were secured, used, kept, and betrayed, as well as their content, can be found in Thucydides' account of the Peloponnesian War. By contrast, at the same time, the worst the Athenian patriots can say of the Spartans is, "Don't you know that to a Spartan, his pledged word, his oath, his solemn sacrifice, counts for nothing?" (Aristophanes. *The Acharnians* 63.)

3. Zuger A, Miles SH. Physicians, AIDS, and occupational risks: Historic traditions and ethical obligations. JAMA 1987;258:1924–8.

4. Herodotus 6:86b.

5. Thucydides 3.83. Similar comments are seen in Plato. *Laws XI:916–7, 937*.

6. Von Staden H. "In a pure and holy way:" Personal and professional conduct in the Hippocratic Oath. J Hist Med Allied Sci 1996;51:406–8.

7. Euripides. *Hippolytus 375–84, 424–6, 486–8, 502–3*.

8. See discussion in the introduction to Chapter 5. It is also a statement that is very different from Pythagorean mysticism, which would be expected if Edelstein's hypothesis were true.

9. Finnell says this passage calls for negative "sanctions" against those who transgress the provisions of the *Oath* (Finnell V. Reforming medicine. Chalcedon Rep 2001;(Jan):426). I disagree. This passage invited future humanity to evaluate physicians without calling down sanctions or divine punishments. Humans in the eternal future would not affect a long-dead physician anyway. This closing is, therefore, an impetration (entreaty), not an imprecation.

Sealey 98–99 discusses how Greek oaths did not assume that the object of the invocation (e.g., the god Apollo) was the agent of judgment. So, Athene or Zeus could have been the agent of judgment and sanction.

10. The *Oresteia* dramatizes the point when the gods tempered the idea of justice as ordained vengeance with a justice that could end destructive cycles of vengeance (Fagles R, Stanford WB, "A Reading of the *Oresteia*: The Serpent and the Eagle," in Aeschylus [1966] 13–97). See also Dodds 141 and Lloyd-Jones 54–103. This drama about contending oaths and loyalties was written about sixty years before the *Oath* at a time of intense turmoil in Athens (Meier 82–149). Athene (Wisdom) proposes that a human conscience, capable of meting out justice with compassion and taking account of remorse, was required to close to socially destructive cycles of justifiable revenge. This shift from justice as "divine revenge" to justice as "psychological guilt" had profound implications for medicine. (Kudlien F. Early Greek primitive medicine. Clio Med 1968;3:305–36. Pearson 90–135.)

11. The most complete argument for this internal morality of medicine is found in Kass 224–246 and Pellegrino. The December 2001 issue of the Journal of Medicine and Philosophy discusses the debate about the internal morality of medicine: Veatch RM, Miller FG. The internal morality of medicine: An introduction. J Med Philos 2001;6:555–7. Pellegrino E. The internal morality of clinical medicine: A paradigm for the ethics of the helping and healing professions. J Med Philos 2001;6:559–79. Miller FG, Brody H. The internal morality of medicine: An evolutionary perspective. J Med Philos 2001;6:581–995. Beauchamp TL. Internal and external standards for medical morality. J Med Philos 2001;6:601–19. Veatch RM. The impossibility of a morality internal to medicine. J Med Philos 2001;6:21–42. Arras

JD. A method in search of a purpose: The internal morality of medicine. J Med Philos 2001;6:643–62. The Center for Clinical Medical Ethics at the Pritzker School of Medicine at the University of Chicago exemplifies this position.

12. Meier 186–221. Nisbet 10–46.

13. Euripides (1958), editor's notes at 70, 122–4. *The Persians*, for example, gives an empathic account of the suffering of these enemies of the Greeks (Aeschylus).

14. Wilkinson T. "Bosnians Recall Karadzic, a Neighbor Turned Enemy." *Los Angeles Times*, July 23, 1995.

15. American College of Physicians. The role of the physician and the medical profession in the prevention of international torture and in the treatment of its survivors. Ann Int Med 1995;122:607–13. Thomsen JL. The role of the pathologist in human rights abuses. J Clin Path 2000;53:569–72; Iacopino V, Heisler M, Pishevar S, Kirschner RH. Physician complicity in misrepresentation and omission of evidence of torture in post-detention medical examinations in Turkey. JAMA 1996;276:396–402. See also British Medical Association.

16. Sorensen B, Vesti P. Medical education for the prevention of torture. Med Educ 1990;24:467–9.

17. His indictment details his actions: http://www.un.org/icty/indictment/english/kar-ii950724e.htm.

18. Go to www.interpol.int and enter the Wanted section, from their search Karadzic. Accessed on July 7, 2002.

19. 48th General Assembly Somerset West, Republic of South Africa, October 1996.

20. See Ahmad K. Human-rights groups express alarm at prosecution of Turkish doctors. Lancet 2000;355(9210):1167.

21. Amnesty International. Medical Letter Writing Action: Prosecution of doctors: Dr H. Zeki Uzun, Turkey index: (07/07/2002). www.web.amnesty.org/ai.nsf/Index/EUR440282000.

AFTERWORD: THE *OATH* FOR OUR TIME

The *Oath's* passages span the history of medicine from its genesis in the age of the Olympian gods to its unfolding judgment by "all human beings for time eternal." The traverse from divine instructors to human appraisal recapitulates the larger narrative of Greek mythology that proceeds from creation epics, to Olympian gods and their heroic offspring who taught justice to humans, and closes with humans' assuming responsibility for a world from which the gods have retreated.[1] The *Oath* was written in the middle of that history. The Greek physicians remembered and still swore by the ancient gods. Olympian oracles still revealed the ancient order, but the gods themselves no longer commingled with humans as they had when Apollo loved Coronis and sired Asclepius. As the *Oath* was written, empirical prediction was replacing divination in medicine, astronomy, and mathematics. Even the analysis of history was becoming a science rather than a discerning of unfolding divine judgments on societies. Thucydides was influenced by the clinical use of eyewitness observations and natural causality in his recounting of the Peloponnesian Wars.[2] Today, history has moved further on; the Greek oracles are silent.

The physicians who swore the *Oath* could not have foreseen the interplay of history and the ethics of medicine. Judaism, Christianity, Islam, and other faiths brought new values to the physician's work. African, Asian, European, and American cultures contributed new theories and understandings about the roles of healers and the ethics of healing. Humankind has rejected slavery and is slowly turning from the subordination of women, institutions that the *Oath* accepted. Western thought engendered a new intellectual endeavor called "medical ethics." Today the *Oath* is one medical ethic in a world of contending and diverse moral systems. If the *Oath* merely memorializes the postulates of ancient Greek medicine (that medicine is a natural science and that being a physician is a moral enterprise), it would be still be a noteworthy relic. I held this minimalist view of its value when I began this exploration. As I came to understand how the *Oath* might have spoken to its own culture, it became easier to see what it might have to say to ours.

Can the *Oath* still speak to our time? Stuart Spicker, a medical ethicist, recently derided a new statement of medical ethics with these words:

> As for oaths of virtually any sort—especially those generated for professionals—they've never directed professional conduct; neither, I suspect, will any contemporary version. Historians of medicine have years ago documented the irrelevancy of the Hippocratic Oath, especially in Hippocrates' own time. More recent literature finds professionals ignoring the precepts altogether.[3]

This harsh and unprovable assessment misapprehends the nature of oaths. Most of us respond to reminders that our lives are evaluated and in some mysterious way fulfilled by acknowledging some standard of moral coherence and purpose. The cautionary words of an oath, a sermon, a play, a friend, or even a stranger may cause us to reflect as we move along paths that are new to us or on those that are so oft-traveled that we have become unmindful of the importance of our steps. In these moments of renewed moral consciousness, we can choose in new ways with a refreshed sense of what is at stake. Oaths do not compel ethical behavior, but they are human instruments that are crafted to sensitize the reader to moral moments and choices. Sometimes, as when Dr. Uzun resisted torture in Turkey, an honored moral voice can serve as an anchor that helps a person stand fast when the tide of history is running strongly in another direction. Many instruments have been devised to articulate the moral nature of being a physician.

VOICE

Medical ethics instruments fall into two large groups: those that require a physician to perform them and those that exhort physicians to act in a certain way.

Oaths and petitionary prayers are examples of those that are written to be read as first-person proclamations of moral commitments.[4] For example, the *Oath* begins, "I swear by Apollo" and proceeds with to articulate its moral positions with "I will" or "I will not." The Physician' Prayer of Moses Maimonides (twelfth-century CE) is a petitionary prayer: "Inspire me with love for my Art and for Thy creatures. Do not allow thirst for profit, ambition for renown and admiration, to interfere with my profession."[5] The Oath of Asaph and Yohanan (sixth-century CE) consists of two parts: rabbinical instructions on what is required of a physician ("Do not harden your heart from pitying the poor and healing the needy") and a responsive proclamation ("We will do all that you exhorted and ordered, for it is a commandment of the Torah, and we must do it with all our hearts, with our soul and with all our might").[6] The 1998 Declaration of Geneva begins: "I solemnly pledge myself. . . ." Reading in a proclamatory voice commits the physician to the avowed promises.

To an increasing degree, the first-person voice of medical oaths is being supplanted by ethical instructions for a physician to study rather than to proclaim. For example, the American Medical Association's Council on Ethical and Judicial Affairs asserts that: "At a minimum, a physician's ethical duties include terminating the physician–patient relationship before initiating a dating, romantic, or sexual relationship with a patient.[7] By contrast, a morally accountable person stands behind a statement like, "I will be far . . . from sexual acts both upon women's bodies and upon men's, both of the free and of the slaves."[8] Governments, international organizations, and professional associations promulgate many such hortatory codes, regulations, declarations, and laws. This voice offers several advantages to institutional sponsors. First, though they may be aimed at physicians, their moral authority rests with the sponsor. This obviates the need to assert a fundamental value for the position in a world where the traditional foundations of moral claims are challenged. In response to the challenge, "Who says physicians should not have sex with patients?" the answer returns: "The AMA's Council on Ethical and Judicial Affairs says so." Second, sponsors may unilaterally define the boundaries of medical ethics. Some asserted boundaries are reasonably grounded in circumscribed expertise. For example, an association of neonatologists might offer an ethics opinion on the moral dilemmas posed by "extracorporeal membrane oxygenators" (a complex machine to oxygenate the blood of critically ill premature infants). Sometimes, however, a medical organization's moral horizon may sunder a moral community. For example, the expansively named "Charter for Medical Professionalism" grounds its vision of medical ethics on the "frustration" of physicians in "industrialized countries."[9] By so doing, this Charter unjustifiably narrows the moral scope of medical professionalism to the parochial priorities of economically and politically privileged physicians and marginalizes the grave economic and human rights issues faced by physicians working in poor or totalitarian nations.

Notwithstanding the increasing number of instruments and the shift to hortatory medical ethics codes, one could argue that the *Oath* is doing better than ever. It was rarely mentioned in Europe until about 1500, when it emerged in the context of Renaissance interest in Greek and Roman civilizations.[10] The percentage of American medical schools reciting an oath increased from twenty-four percent in 1928 to seventy-two percent in 1958, and to ninety-eight percent by 1993.[11] Half of these schools use a variant of the Hippocratic *Oath*; the rest use other texts. Even so, only a handful of schools expose students to the text of the *Oath* during their medical ethics education.[12] One might speculate that the use of the oath format reflects an unmet hunger for sacred ceremonies. This may be partly true, but I think that oaths endure because they require the physicians to speak of their values. At some level, physicians recognize that a personal revelation of moral commitments is necessary to the practice of medicine.

In a chapter entitled "The Patient Examines the Doctor," Anatole Broyard describes his search for an urologist to treat his newly diagnosed prostate cancer, a disease that had taken his father's life. Mr. Broyard was escorted into an urologist's office that he approvingly noted was fitted with books, well-chosen antiques, and signs of the physician's family and hobby. Mr. Broyard took this evidence of the physician's passions as signs that he "knew how to live and, by extension, how to look after the lives of others." Unfortunately, another doctor came in and said, "Let's go to my office." The second physician's office and demeanor was "modern and anonymous," and the new doctor had "no sign of a tragic sense of life."[13] That physician's moral anonymity eventually led Broyard to seek another physician. What do we know about physician–patient relationships and the personal revelations of ancient Greek physicians?

Greek physicians wrote intensely personal case records. Many examples have been cited; here is another one, in this case from *Epidemics I*:

Silenius lived on Broadway near the place of Eualcidas. After over-exertion, drinking, and exercise at the wrong time he was attacked by fever. . . . Third day: General exacerbation . . . no sleep at night; much rambling, laughter, singing; no power of restraining himself.[14]

The personal details of this case speak of a human relationship between the physician and patient. The physician knew where Silenius lived, his neighbors, his work, his drinking. The physician did not simply record delirium; he reported rambling speech, laughter, and singing, and discreetly noted a certain lack of decorum. Though Greek medicine insisted on objective observation, doctoring was still the encounter of one person with another.

Modern medicine seems to be at risk of losing this blend of objectivity and relationship. In some medical records, the patient as a person nearly disappears into jargon and measurements. It is common to find records that go like this: "65 yo wm. CC: DOE, orthopnea. PI: $\emptyset$ CP, $\uparrow$15 # in 3 mo. RF: HBP, $\uparrow$chol, DM. PMH: CHF with EF 25%."[15] In one disquieting study, only a third of resident physicians knew whether their adult patients had children.[16] Public discontent with medicine is partly grounded on how the physician–patient relationship increasingly resembles an encounter between a technician and a malfunctioning machine.[17]

People encounter each other through dialogue. We know that Greek physicians advertised their education, publicly demonstrated their skill, and sought to promote their reputation by word of mouth. The *Oath* resembled other ancient medical treatises in that it discusses how to practice good medicine and to honor one's colleagues and treat patients with decorum. It was unique, however, in requiring the reader to use the proclamatory voice. This first-person voice obliged the physician to speak and reveal his personal commitments. As Broyard noted, the patient's trust rests on more than credentialed assurances of a physician's skill; it also rests on the patient's confidence in how this particular physician (of all those who are comparably skilled) will use the tools and respect the intimacy of a clinical relationship. In selecting the first-person voice for the *Oath*, its authors explicitly spoke of the necessity for each physician to reveal his professional moral commitments. The first-person voice may be part of the energy behind the *Oath*'s endurance.

By reading a set of statements that begin "I will . . . " and "I will not . . . " a physician is put in a position where she or he must, at some level, accept, reject, interpret, or amend the vow. In this interpretation, the physician reflects on his or her own experience, values, medical practice, and culture. The *Oath's* words like "injustice" are, or should be, read in light of what these words have come to mean in a culture scarred by racism and where countless people cannot afford basic health care. Through the first-person proclamatory voice, the *Oath* reinvents its meaning. This is also why it must be studied rather than simply brought out for ritual use. A modern reader needs help to read words like "Apollo" or "holy." The *Oath* can teach if we read it in the third person to try to understand its message before we read it again to proclaim its meaning for medical ethics in our time. The *Oath's* first-person voice reflects a belief that medical ethics must be pledged and lived rather than merely codified and taught.

AUTHORITY

What does the *Oath* teach the diaspora of modern medical cultures? Its authority in its own time is unknown. For the last five hundred years, Western Christian culture has molded the *Oath*, especially its abortion and euthanasia passages, to buttress moral conclusions formed long after the *Oath* was written. Until 1940, when Edelstein dismissed Greek medical ethics as mere decorum and attributed the *Oath* to Pythagoreans, it had been assumed that it represented a point of view from the ancient Greek medical community. Today, its authority appears to be greater in European than in Asian medical cultures.[18] Jewish institutions and professionals tend to prefer oaths by members of their own faith. In the West, the *Oath's* core message is still powerful. Medicine is a moral enterprise upheld by personal moral commitment (the proclamatory voice) and integrity ("In a pure and holy way, I will guard my life and *techné*"). Physicians must share medical knowledge, benefit the ill, and promote justice. Though this core still has lessons to teach, the *Oath's* examples seem to be more culturally conditioned.

It is interesting that the body of the *Oath* is structured as principles and examples rather than as a list of commandments (see "Introduction," Part II). The principles are the two uses of "benefit and justice," and they constitute the moral core of the *Oath*. The examples are contingent both with regard to the culture of ancient Greece and to the evolving understanding of the principles, as shall be discussed later. The four examples are:

I will not give a drug that is deadly to anyone if asked for it, nor will I suggest the way to such a counsel.

I will not give a woman a destructive pessary.

[I will refrain] from sexual acts both upon women's bodies and upon men's, both of the free and of the slaves.

I will remain silent about whatever I may see or hear in or even outside of treatment, holding things that should not ever be blurted out outside to be unutterable.

Preceding chapters on these examples have discussed the cultural changes that diminish our ability to simply take these examples as the *Oath's* message to the medical ethics of our time. Greece was a highly patriarchal society. The *Oath's* restriction of medical education to men may be set side without dethroning its principles of justice and beneficence. The vow on sexual relations tacitly accepts the legitimacy of slavery. The provision on confidentiality did not envision the complexities of information systems in the modern health-care system, including issues like insurance, workers' compensation, the duty to warn, and the moral autonomy of minors. The passages on deadly drugs or abortion are not the *Oath's* moral axis, and they are abused when they are seen as ancient ratifications of moral arguments against euthanasia, physician-assisted suicide, or abortion that arose long after the *Oath's* time. These examples illustrate the difficulty in abstracting moral advice from one culture and applying it to another. This difficulty does not, however, justify discounting the *Oath's* lessons for medical ethics in our time.

Indeed, one of the ironies of the *Oath's* contemporary reception is how the debate about its examples has eclipsed the examination of its core message. For example, the recruitment of its passage on destructive pessaries into the framework of the modern abortion debate has led many schools and even prominent ethicists[19] to excise, rather than to examine the historical setting of, these words. The very persons who misused the passage in the first place then take such excisions as confirming the moral decline of medicine. Through such misuse, a relationship with an important document about medical ethics is being lost.

The content of the *Oath* speaks to three critical issues in the ethics of medicine. Who are you as a physician? To what are you committed? To what are you accountable? Each generation of physicians confronts these questions and arrives at their own answers. The *Oath* can still help us answer each of them.

WHO ARE PHYSICIANS?

This ethics question looks at the moral underpinnings of the profession, the identities of its practitioners, and their duties to secure the profession's future. The *Oath's* Apollonian opening refers to a rich set of moral stories about the foundation of medicine. These stories say that being a healer is a heroic enterprise. They tell of how the passion to heal is grounded on love and grief and teach that physicians must not pretend to contest the fact of human mortality. Asclepius, "Unceasingly gentle," and Epione, "Soothing," passed a common spirit to the diverse branches of healing. Physicians swore by the entire family of Asclepius and Epione. The *Oath* explicitly mentioned Hygieia (goddess of health or preventive health care) and Panacea (All-Heal, goddess of remedies) and called on their siblings, "all the gods as well as goddesses" as well. In this way, physicians embraced Iaso (goddess of medicine), Aigle (radiance) and Telesphorus (god of convalescence). In opening medical apprenticeships to sons from all families, the *Oath* departed from the hereditary Asclepiads to make each practitioner, teacher, and student a part of this family. This two-fold opening of the medical family to the extended family of Aclepius and Epione and outside the literal descendents of physicians contains several lessons for modern medical ethics.

First, it invites us to reconceptualize medical ethics in a multidisciplinary health-care system. Health care is increasingly a multidisciplinary affair.[20] There are epidemiologists and public officials—the descendents of Hygieia.[21] There are pharmacists, formulary committees, pharmaceutical companies, and public bodies that allocate funds to develop new therapies—the descendents of Panacea. Those who specialize in recovery, rehabilitation, and convalescence are descendents of Telesphorus. Those who use the healing sciences to soothe, nurses' aides, are descendents of Epione. Nurses and physician's assistants may properly be named descendents of Iaso. The descendents of Aigle restore a radiant countenance to those who suffer: nutritionists, hospice workers, and home health-care aides. All of these healers are descendents of Aclepius and Epione. The written records of multidisciplinary care in ancient Greece do not do justice to what appears to have actually occurred. The scant records that are available refer to physicians working with male and female medical and surgical assistants, nurses, and midwives.[22] Greek physicians recorded and began the process of validating the oral lore root healers.

From the *Oath's* moral metaphor of a family of medicine, we could take a cue to be more receptive to embracing a family metaphor as an alternative to the physician-centered hierarchy. This would take us to a more unified ethic for multidisciplinary team care.[23] It would mean more than ceasing empirically unsupported turf battles between physicians and nurse-practitioners, optometrists, or psychologists over prescribing privileges and the like. It would suggest more aggressively moving to collaborative practice models with a more balanced sharing of authority, accountability, and reimbursement insofar as they can be shown to improve health-care delivery.

Second, academic medicine can take a cue from the opening of the Asclepian family to dismantle the quasi-hereditary race- and class-based barriers to medical training that unjustly diminish the numbers of healers from African American, Native American, and other minority communities.[24] Healers from more diverse communities are more likely to effectively advocate on behalf of correcting the forces that are causing these communities to experience under-treatment and unacceptably poor health-care outcomes, speak languages that are underrepresented in the health-care system, and treat persons from under-served populations.[25] The medical schools should be opened just as the Asclepian family of practitioners was opened 2,400 years ago.

Third, in its vows to sustain teachers and to impart "rules, lectures, and all the rest of learning," the *Oath* says that the integrity of the teaching enterprise is critical to the survival of the medical profession. It is ironic that the ethics of medical education is now largely confined to matters such as sexual relations between faculty and students and various forms of academic discrimination. The *Oath* points us to consider the integrity of research and the dissemination of information.

Finally, it is noteworthy that as the *Oath* honors the house of healers, it repeatedly cautions us as well. It refers to failures of ability. It speaks of the need to guard one's integrity and refers to the temptation to blur, confound, and transgress. Its specific injunctions, such as sexual relations with patients, presumably allude to abuses witnessed by Greek physicians. The *Oath* does not simply glorify healers. Medical ethics today is sometimes an overly sunny recounting of physicians' aspirations and accomplishments. Since *Oath* was written, there have been many sobering examples of healers who have sold these aspirations short or who have put medicine to evil purposes. As we lift up and honor the ethics and heroes of medicine, we must, as the *Oath* does, remember those who misused medicine to fortify racism,[26] justify genocide,[27] torture, supervise executions, and work to turn diseases into weapons.[28]

TO WHAT ARE YOU COMMITTED?

The medical ethics of the *Oath* are centered on two principles, beneficence and justice, that are anchored in and lived through the integrity of the physician. It offers four examples of the application of these principles for medical practice: the disavowals of deadly drugs, destructive pessaries, sexual relations in the course of clinical care, and indiscreet speech. By this structure, the *Oath* suggests that the form of medical ethics should include principles and topics that are arranged to address the societal and clinical roles of the healer. In taking this lead from the *Oath*, we can move to consider what it specifically offers us as we fashion a medical ethics for our time.

Principles first: The *Oath* notably promotes the principles of beneficence and justice twice, deploying in two different directions. The first looks outward, for the benefit of the ill and to keep them from injustice. This pertains to the role of the physician as promoting health in society and engaging in matters of public health, human rights, and harmful ecological change.[29] The principles are employed a second time, in this case in a vow to benefit the ill while keeping far from all voluntary and destructive injustice. This ethic looks inward to the physician's conduct of the clinical relationship. These principles are still serviceable though contemporary ethics has added a new one: respect for a patient's autonomy.

Respect for autonomy, though well entrenched in the United States, differs from how the *Oath* used "beneficence" and "justice" in several respects. It came into being in medical ethics as a principle of protest.[30] In this sense, it tempered an internal medical ethic that had become disrespectful of a changing cultural climate. The abuses that led to this principle's being articulated for medicine included: performing harmful research without consent; not informing patients of the truth of their diseases; the sterilization of African Americans; the empirically unjustified use of restraints, psychosurgery, or psychoactive drugs on persons who were institutionalized; the performance of mastectomies on anesthetized women who had consented only to biopsies; refusing to per-form abortions without a husband's consent or without permission by hospital medical morals committee; rejecting patients' choice to choose loved ones as they wished, and so on. A second difference between autonomy and the prin-ciples of beneficence and justice as those two latter principles are used in the *Oath* is that the former mostly applies to clinical ethics. For example, respect for autonomy has been applied to the right to refuse a proposed standard of care (and even the right to demand futile treatments), but not to the social right of a person to secure adequate health care. Pellegrino and Thomasma argue that beneficence should have been enough to encompass respect for persons or autonomy.[31] Perhaps it might have been, if medical ethics had kept updat-ing the examples it used to illustrate its core principles.

It is admirable that the *Oath* offered topical examples of the application of its principles. These must have illustrated particularly vexing issues for the physicians or society of that time. By offering examples and by holding itself up to the judgment of history, the *Oath* suggests that the fear that an example might be of topical or temporary concern should not confine medical ethics. I agree. Medical ethics is inherently topical. Topical ethics work, like that of Rheinhold Neibuhr, can instruct a culture even though it quickly passes into history. Physician homicide was an issue in ancient Greece. Physician-assisted euthanasia or executions are important issues today. The modern concern may be addressed without pretending that the *Oath's* disavowal of deadly drugs spoke of them. Furthermore, the *Oath* does not suggest that deadly drugs, abortive pessaries, sex with patients, and indiscreet speech delimit some conceptual corral of all the topics of medical ethics. Given the freedom to select our own examples to illustrate the principles of medical ethics, what examples might we choose?

The physicians of ancient Greece did not envision many of the ethical di-lemmas that would confront the modern physician. Many of the topics in the headlines will not involve very many lives. These include the clinical topics of cloning, custody fights over frozen embryos, and even euthanasia. The grand-est challenges of our time are posed by the financing of health care. Even Prometheus did not grant foresight into the ethical dilemmas of capitated re-imbursement in managed care,[32] the unbearable expense of health technolo-gies in the Third World, or universal access to health care.[33] Such matters are deservedly addressed as examples of the physician's commitment to fundamen-tal principles for clinical and social ethics. How might this be done?

Today, all economically developed nations whose healers claim descent from the Hippocratic tradition view universal access to affordable health care as a moral obligation of their health care system—every developed nation except the United States. Many U.S. physicians argue that universal access to basic health care is about societal or political values that are external to medical ethics, and certainly outside the vision of the *Oath*. I believe that physicians could embrace a commitment to working for affordable universal health care as exemplifying the principle "from what is to their harm or injustice I will keep them." This societal example could be answered with a clinical example of "how to remain far from destructive injustice" as physicians considered the stewardship of resources that would be required to achieve just access to health care. By this example, physicians would take a giant step toward resolving the paradox of U.S. medicine in which trust in physicians is waning as the bounty of healing technologies multiplies.

IN WHAT WAY ARE YOU ACCOUNTABLE?

The words that invite "all human beings for time eternal" assert that the past is to be remembered, not idolized.[34] It invites debate, not veneration. Each physician is thus obliged to make a commitment to the ethics of medicine in light of the lessons of the past, the problems of our time, and the judgment of those who follow us. Just as the ancient Greek physicians did with the medical lore that they received, we receive this text along with the rest of medical knowledge as a human compilation of wisdom to improve upon as we, in turn, pass our conclusions for evaluation by all human beings for time eternal.

NOTES

1. Calasso 386–91. Aeschylus, *Oresteia*.

2. Hanson VD. Introduction in *Thucydides xii*.

3. Message on Medical College of Wisconsin Bioethics Discussions, e-mail chat line. Feb. 8, 2002 (used with permission of author).

4. Sulmasy DP. What is an oath and why should a physician swear one? Theoret Med & Bioethics 1999;20:329–46. Hasday LR. The Hippocratic Oath as literary text: A dialogue between law and medicine. Yale J Health Policy, Law, Ethics 2002;II(2): 299–323.

5. Rosner F. The physician's prayer attributed to Moses Maimonides. Bull Hist Med 1967;41:440–54.

6. Shlomo P. "The Oath of Asaph the Physician and Yohanan Ben Zabda. Its Relation to the Hippocratic Oath and the Doctrina Duarum Viarum of the Didache." Proceedings of the Israel Academy of Science and Humanities 1975;9:223–64.

7. E-8.14 "Sexual Misconduct in the Practice of Medicine," in 1992 Code of Ethics: Annotated Current Opinions. Chicago, IL: American Medical Association, 1992.

8. Examples of this difference are easy to see. For example, the *Oath* says, "In a pure and holy way, I will guard my life and my art and science," whereas a recent document in the instructional voice says, "The profession is responsible for the integrity of this knowledge, which is based on scientific evidence and physician experience." American Board of Internal Medicine Foundation, et al., op. cit. See also the World Medical Organization. Declaration of Helsinki. BMJ 1996;313(7070): 1448–9.

9. American Board of Internal Medicine Foundation, American College of Physicians–American Society of Internal Medicine Foundation, and European Federations of Internal Medicine. Medical Professionalism in the New Millennium: A Physicians Charter. Ann Intern Med 2002;136:243–6.

10. Nutton V. What's in an oath? J R Coll Physicians in Lond 1995;29:518–24.

11. Friedlander WJ. Oaths given by U.S. and Canadian medical schools. Soc Sci & Med 1982;16:115–20. Carey EJ. The formal use of the Hippocratic Oath for medical students at commencement exercises. Bull Assn Amer Med Coll 1928;159–66. Irish DP, McMurray DW. Professional oaths and American medical colleges. J Chronic Disease 1965;18:275–89. Orr RD, Pang N, Pellegrino ED, Siegler M. Use of the Hippocratic Oath: A review of twentieth-century practice and a content analysis of oaths administered in medical schools in the U.S. and Canada in 1993. J Clin Ethics 1997;8(winter):374–5.

12. Dubois JM, Burkemper H. Ethics education in U.S. medical schools: A study of syllabi. Acad Med 2002;77:432–37.

13. Broyard 31–58.

14. *Epidemics I, fourteen cases: case II.*

15. Translated, this reads: 65 yo wm [65-year-old white male]: CC [Chief complaint]: DOE, orthopnea [dyspnea on exertion and shortness of breath unless sitting up in a chair]. PI [Present illness]: $\emptyset$ CP [chest pain], ↑15 #s in 3 mo [months]. RF [risk factors]: HBP [high blood pressure], ↑chol [high cholesterol], DM [diabetes]. PMH [Past medical history]: CHF with EF 25% [congestive heart failure with a machine measured heart function of 25% with a normal of 75%].

16. Griffith CH, Rich EC, Wilson JF. Housestaff's knowledge of their patients' social histories. Acad Med 1995;70:64–6.

17. Broyard. Mishler. Shorter.

18. See Temkin. Also, a forthcoming book examines the historical reinvention of Hippocrates and Greek medicine (Cantor).

19. Pellegrino and Thomasma 206.

20. Druss BG, Marcus SC, Olfson M, et al. Trends in care by nonphysician clinicians in the United States. N Engl J Med 2003;348:130–7. Aiken LH. Achieving an interdisciplinary workforce in health care. N Engl J Med 2003 348;164–6.

21. The authority of Hygiea and public health and the principles of "benefiting the ill" and "keeping them from injustice" might also extend to medical ethics with regard to the healers' role in promoting responsible social policies, even such long-term threats to the ecosystem such as global warming (Jonas).

22. See chapters 7 and 9.

23. Purtilo RB. Rethinking the ethics of confidentiality and health-care teams. Bioethics Forum. 1998;14(3–4):23–7. Browne A, Carpenter C, Cooledge C, et al. Bridging the professions: An integrated and interdisciplinary approach to teaching health care ethics. Acad Med 1995;70:1002–5. May T. The nurse under physician authority. J Med Ethics 1993;19:223–9. Joseph MV, Conrad AP. Social work influence on interdisciplinary ethical decision making in health care settings. Health Soc Work 1989;14:22–30. Irvine R, Kerridge I, McPhee J, Freeman S. Interprofessionalism and ethics: consensus or clash of cultures? J Interprofess Care 2002;16:199–210. Mularski RA, Bascom P, Osborne ML. Educational agendas for interdisciplinary end-of-life curricula. Crit Care Med 2001;29(2 Suppl):N16–23.

24. Barzansky B, Jonas HS, Etzel SI. Educational programs in U.S. medical schools 1999–2000. JAMA 2000;284:1114–20.

25. Institute of Medicine.

26. Graves (2001). Gould. Jones (1981).

27. Proctor.

28. Anonymous. Chemical and biological weaponry and war. Ann Intern Med 1969;71:204–8. Christopher GW, Cieslak TJ, Pavlin JA, Eitzen EM. Biological warfare: A historical perspective. JAMA 1997;278:412–7. JAMA 1997;278:412–7. Gellert GA. Global health interdependence and the international physicians' movement. JAMA 1990;264:610–3.

29. The social ethic of medicine extends to health-harming effects of the increasing gap between the world's richest nations and its poorest (Gellert GA. Global health interdependence and the international physicians' movement. JAMA 1990;264:610–3), the healers' role in teaching and promoting responsible social policies for threats to the ecosystem such as ozone depletion or global warming (Jonas), human rights, weapons of mass destruction (Chemical and biological weaponry and war. Ann Intern Med 1969;71:204–8). Christopher GW, Cieslak TJ, Pavlin JA, Eitzen EM. Bio-

logical warfare. A historical perspective. JAMA 1997;278:412–7. Forrow L, Sidel VW. Medicine and nuclear war: From Hiroshima to mutual assured destruction to abolition 2000. JAMA 1998;280:456–61), torture, and economic sanctions (Morin K, Miles SH, for the American College of Physicians. Economic sanctions and professional ethics. Ann Intern Med 2000;132:158–61).

    30. Fletcher. Jonsen (1998) 335–8.

    31. Pellegrino and Thomasma.

    32. A full discussion of the ethics of managed care goes far outside the scope of this book. A few suggestions are: Hall MA, Berenson RA. Ethical practice in managed care: A dose of realism. Ann Intern Med 1998;128:395–402. Jecker NS. Managed competition and managed care: What are the ethical issues? Clin Geriatr Med 1994;10:527–40. LeBlang TR. Informed consent and disclosure in the physician–patient relationship: Expanding obligations for physicians in the United States. Med Law 1995;14:429–44.

    33. Churchill.

    34. Nisbet 10–46.

APPENDIX A: TIMELINE

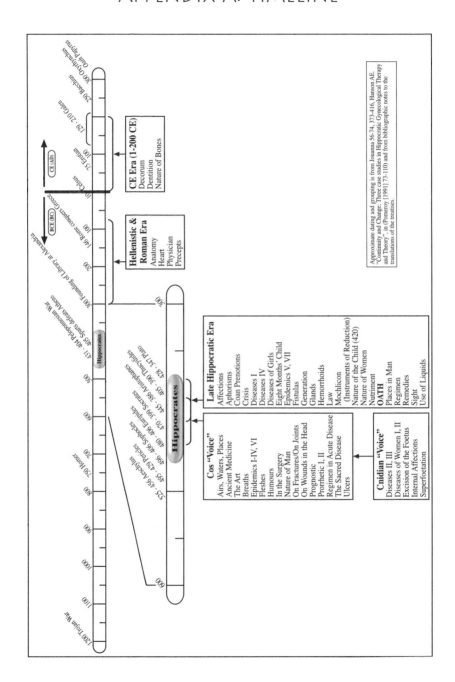

Cos "Voice"
Airs, Waters, Places
Ancient Medicine
The Art
Breaths
Epidemics I–IV, VI
Fleshes
Humours
In the Surgery
Nature of Man
On Fractures/On Joints
On Wounds in the Head
Prognostic
Prorrhetic I, II
Regimen in Acute Disease
The Sacred Disease
Ulcers

Late Hippocratic Era
Affections
Aphorisms
Coan Prenotions
Crisis
Diseases I
Diseases IV
Diseases of Girls
Eight Months' Child
Epidemics V, VII
Fistulas
Generation
Glands
Hemorrhoids
Law
Mochlicon
(Instruments of Reduction)
Nature of the Child (420)
Nature of Women
Nutriment
OATH
Places in Man
Regimen
Remedies
Sight
Use of Liquids

Cnidian "Voice"
Diseases II, III
Diseases of Women I, II
Excision of the Foetus
Internal Affections
Superfoetation

Hellenistic & Roman Era
Anatomy
Heart
Physician
Precepts

CE Era (1–200 CE)
Decorum
Dentition
Nature of Bones

Approximate dating and grouping is from Jouanna 56–74, 373–416, Hanson AE. "Continuity and Change: Three case studies in Hippocratic Gynecological Therapy and Theory", in (Pomeroy [1991] 73–110) and from bibliographic notes to the translations of the treatises.

187

APPENDIX B: THE *OATH* AS A CURRICULAR OUTLINE FOR MEDICAL ETHICS

The *Oath* is widely used in graduation ceremonies either at the end of medical school or at the beginning of clinical clerkships during medical school. Such ceremonies are often the first and last time that a student will encounter this text.[1] Exclusively ceremonial use diminishes the value of the *Oath* in those ceremonies and forgoes an opportunity to employ this fascinating text in teaching medical ethics.[2] The *Oath* can serve as a coherent starting point and organizing framework for a curriculum in medical ethics.

There is no self-evident way to organize a medical ethics curriculum. There are problems with trying to fit a curriculum in the order from conception to death or on expanding circles of social organization (e.g., patient, physician, physician–patient relationship, health care institutions, medicine in society). The ordinal principles of autonomy, justice, and beneficence are too rigid for the complexity of narrative ethics or casuistry. Social critiques, including feminist insights into medicine, are also essential and further complicate the task for a teacher who would attempt to assert one tidy, unifying conceptual organization of the field.

The *Oath*'s passages and the structure of its argument are arguably more engaging and no less serviceable than any other proposed curriculum. It need not be a procrustean bed for a curriculum, though I believe that it can be used as an outline. Table APP–B.1 shows how the *Oath* might be used as a framework for a medical ethics course. Its short text certainly does not adequately explicate the nuances of medical ethics for its time or ours. I emphasize that this topical outline does not commend a particular didactic method. Small group discussions, case analysis, literary readings, lectures, presentations by patients, and practical demonstrations or examinations with model patients, all have a role to play at various times in medical ethics education. A full discussion of the pedagogy of Medical Ethics goes far beyond the scope of this book.

The topical content and depth of medical ethics education remain a matter of debate.[3] It will vary for various health professions and according to when ethics education occurs during the degree program. Time may not permit including all of the suggested "curricular topics." It does seem wise, however, to cover some less-conventional topics so that students can learn how to generalize from the familiar to the less common. This will be a necessary skill as new ethical problems present themselves during their careers.

Table APP-B.1. The *Oath* as a Curricular Outline in Medical Ethics

Section of the Oath	Curricular Topics
ORIGINS	
I swear by Apollo the Physician and by Asclepius and by Health and Panacea and by all the gods as well as goddesses, making them judges [witnesses], to bring the following oath and written covenant to fulfillment, in accordance with my power and my judgment;	Medical professionalism and the meaning of making a commitment to be a physician The difference between practicing ethical medicine in a pluralistic society and being a physician with strongly held personal moral or religious or values
TEACHERS	
To regard him who has taught me this *techné* as equal to my parents, and to share, in partnership, my livelihood with him,	Medicine as a guild and authority
LEARNERS	
and to give a share both of rules and of lectures, and of all the rest of learning, to my sons and to the [sons] of him who has taught me and to the pupils who have . . . sworn by a medical convention but by no other.	The responsibilities of physicians in training The responsibility and ethics of research and of sharing noteworthy medical observations (such as adverse medical events) Corporate influences on medical training

Table APP-B.1. (*continued*)

	PUBLIC HEALTH
I will use regimens for the benefit of the ill in accordance with my ability and my judgment, but from [what is] to their harm or injustice I will keep [them].	Justice in health care Access to health care, the uninsured, free care, Good Samaritan laws Public health ethics
	END-OF-LIFE CARE
I will not give a drug that is deadly to anyone if asked [for it], nor will I suggest the way to such a counsel.	Forgoing life-sustaining treatment Euthanasia, physician-assisted suicide, double effect, terminal sedation Brain death Futility Quality-of-life judgments Palliative care, hospice
	REPRODUCTIVE HEALTH CARE
And likewise I will not give a woman a destructive pessary.	Reproductive health care, abortion, assisted reproduction Conscientious objection to patients' choices Emancipated minors
	INTEGRITY
In a pure and holy way I will guard my life and my *techné*.	Integrity and conflicts of interests Industry–physician relations Dual-loyalty problems in managed care, research, occupational medicine, correctional health care, and military medicine
	MEDICAL ERROR
I will not cut, and certainly not those suffering from stone, but I will cede [this] to men [who are] practitioners of this activity.	Managing uncertainty, risk, error, mistakes When and how to use consultants (including ethics consultants)
	CONSENT AND TRUTH-TELLING
Into as many houses as I may enter, I will go for the benefit of the ill,	Physician–patient relationship Beneficence Paternalism Respect for autonomy, informed consent, truth-telling, and disclosing bad news Competence, and persons without decision-making capacity

Table APP-B.1. The *Oath* as a Curricular Outline in Medical Ethics (*continued*)

	Pediatric care
	Alternative medicine and non-validated therapies
	EXPLOITING PATIENTS
while being far from all voluntary and destructive injustice, especially from sexual acts both upon women's bodies and upon men's, both of the free and of the slaves.	The impaired physician
	Boundary violations
	Impact of race, social class, and cultural difference on clinical decision-making
	DISCRETION IN SPEECH
About whatever I may see or hear in treatment, or even without treatment, in the life of human beings—things that should not ever be blurted out outside—I will remain silent, holding such things to be unutterable [sacred, not to be divulged].	Confidentiality, privacy
	Web, mail, e-mail, and leaving telephone messages
	Authorized release of information and physician–employer or physician–insurer communication
	A TRUSTWORTHY PHYSICIAN
If I render this oath fulfilled, and if I do not blur and confound it [making it to no effect] may it be [granted] to me to enjoy the benefits both of life and of *techné*, being held in good repute among all human beings for time eternal. If, however, I transgress and perjure myself, the opposite of these.	Accountability in medicine
	Malpractice, negligence, criminal liability
	Peer review, medical boards
	Physicians and human rights

NOTES

1. Veatch RM. White coat ceremonies: A second opinion. J Med Ethics 2002; 28:5–9.

2. Pearlman RA. The value of an oath of professional conduct: Process, content, or both? J Clin Ethics 1990;1:292–3.

3. Dubois JM, Burkemper H. Ethics education in U.S. medical schools: A study of syllabi. Acad Med 2002;77:432–37. Silverberg LI. Survey of medical ethics in U.S. medical schools: A descriptive study. J Am Osteopath Assoc 2000;100:373–78. Musick DW. Teaching medical ethics: A review of the literature from North American medical schools with emphasis on education. Med, Health Care, Phibsophy 1999;2:239–54. Miles SH, Lane LW, Bickel J, Walker R, Cassel CK. Medical ethics education: Coming of age. Acad Med 1989;64:705–14.

BIBLIOGRAPHY

I consulted a diverse set of books and articles while writing this work. In general the works were of several types. There were ancient Greek works of philosophy, drama, and medicine; modern scholarly work on Greek culture; and modern bioethics works. Excerpts from Greek dramas were used only to illustrate points made by Greek cultural scholars. I used Graves as a primary reference on Greek mythology but relied on Calasso for conveying the narrative sweep of Greek mythology. Books are cited in this appendix because many of them were cited several times. The articles are cited in the endnotes. When multiple translations of ancient texts were available, I tended to use the more recent translation as being more up-to-date and also somewhat clearer, provided that scholarly sources regarded the translation highly.

Choosing among the many translations of the *Oath* is difficult. Three translations stand out on the basis of the authority of their translators: Jones' from 1923, Chadwick and Mann's from 1950, and von Staden's 1996 translation.[1] I elected to use von Staden's version as the primary source for this work because his later work is best positioned to take advantage of recent scholarship in Greek thought. Though the authority of von Staden's translation of the words is unchallengeable, his sentences are prolix. The *Oath* was meant to be spoken aloud, as indeed it often is today. Von Staden acknowledges that the parsing of the *Oath* is, in itself, an act of interpretation. I hope that an equally competent translation that chooses and measures the words for their poetry will be forthcoming.

I focused on the ancient medical treatises that were most contemporary with the *Oath*. These works contain a wealth of material detailing medical practice at the time the *Oath* was written. Unfortunately, portions of the gynecological treatises of ancient Greece are not fully translated into English yet; a forthcoming Loeb translation will remedy this neglect. The customarily cited works on medical ethics, *Decorum* and *Precepts*, were written centuries after the *Oath*. For this reason, I did not draw on them as heavily as have other authors. In that the physicians of ancient Greece were men, I have used male pronouns when writing about them; I then shifted to gender-inclusive pronouns when writing about contemporary cases.

Except where otherwise stated, the Loeb Classical Library translations of the Hippocratic medical treatises are the source for endnote citations. I used newer, well-regarded translations when subsequent scholarship had shown inaccuracies in the older Loeb translations, or when the wording rang truer to the modern ear. The titles of the ancient medical treatises are given in italics. In endnotes, the title of the treatise is followed by the chapter, paragraph, and line numbers as they are assigned to the English text by the translator: e.g., *Epidemics III:14–16* for *Epidemics*, volume 3, lines 14–16.

A three-part list of the cited Hippocratic works follows this paragraph. The first part is the Loeb Classical Library Series. The second part includes translations of treatises that are not in the Loeb series. The third part is a unified listing of all the treatises. This last list takes into account the potentially confusing diversity of titles for the same works. Complete bibliographical information for all books cited in the endnotes follows the translations of the ancient Greek documents.

LOEB SERIES

1. Hippocrates. *Ancient Medicine. Airs, Waters, Places. Epidemics I, III. The Oath. Precepts. Nutriment.* Trans. WHS Jones. Volume I. Cambridge: Loeb Classical Library, 1923a.
2. Hippocrates. *Prognostic. Regimen in Acute Diseases. The Sacred Disease. The Art. Breaths. Law. Decorum. Physician (Chap. I). Dentition.* Trans. WHS Jones. Volume II. Cambridge: Loeb Classical Library, 1923b.

3. Hippocrates. *On Wounds in the Head. In the Surgery. Fractures. Joints, Mochlicon (Instruments of Reduction)*. Trans. ET Withington. Volume III. Cambridge: Loeb Classical Library, 1928.

4. Hippocrates. *Nature of Man. Regimen in Health. Humours. Aphorisms. Regimen I–III. Dreams. Heracleitus: On the Universe*. Trans. WHS Jones. Volume IV. Cambridge: Loeb Classical Library, 1931.

5. Hippocrates. *Affections. Diseases I–II*. Trans. P Potter. Volume V. Cambridge: Loeb Classical Library, 1988.

6. Hippocrates. *Diseases III. Internal Affections. Regimen in Acute Diseases (Appendix)*. Trans. P Potter. Volume VI. Cambridge: Loeb Classical Library, 1988.

7. Hippocrates. *Epidemics II, IV–VII*. Trans. WD Smith. Volume VII. Cambridge: Loeb Classical Library, 1994.

8. Hippocrates. *Places in Man. Glands. Fleshes. Prorrhetic I–II. Physician. Use of Liquids. Ulcers. Haemorrhoids. Fistulas*. Trans. P Potter. Volume VIII. Cambridge: Loeb Classical Library, 1995.

MEDICAL TREATISES PUBLISHED IN OTHER SOURCES

NOTE: Diverse titles given to the same work can be confusing. Where the sources in the following list use titles that differ from the titles in the Loeb series, the Loeb title is given in brackets after the title as it appears in the cited work. For example, if the Loeb volume translated a title as *Law* and one of these sources titled it *Canon*, the cite in the following list would read *Canon* [= *Law*]. A unified index of all the titles follows:

9. Hippocrates. *Places in Man*. Trans. EM Craik. Oxford: Clarendon Press, 1998.

10. Craik EM. *The Hippocratic Treatise: On Anatomy*. Classical Quarterly 1998; 48(i):135–67.

11. Hippocrates. *Diseases of Women I* [a partial translation]. Trans. AE Hanson. Signs: Journal of Women in Culture and Society 1975;1(2):567–584.

12. Hippocrates. *Hippocratic Writings*. (Contains *Oath; Canon* [= *Law*]; *Tradition in Medicine* [= *Ancient Medicine*]; *Epidemics I; Epidemics III; The Science of Medicine* [= *The Art*]; *Airs, Waters, Places; Prognosis* [= *Prognostic*]; *Aphorisms; The Sacred Disease; Dreams; The Nature of Man; A Regimen for Health; Fractures; Seed* [= *On Generation*]; *Nature of the Child; Heart*. Ed. GER Lloyd. Trans. J Chadwick, WN Mann, ET Withington, IM Lonie. London: Penguin Classics, 1950.

13. *Hippocrates: On Head Wounds*. Trans. M Hanson. Bad Langensalza (Germany): Akademie Verlag, 1999.

14. *Oeuvres complètes d'Hippocrate: traduction nouvelle avec le texte Grec en regard.* 10 vols, J B Ballière, Paris, 1839–1861. Trans (into French) E Littré. Reprinted Amsterdam: Hakkert Publishing, 1961–1962. (N.b. I use the Hakkert pagination.)

15. Hippocrates. *The Hippocratic Treatises: On Generation, On the Nature of the Child, Diseases IV.* Trans. IM Lonie. New York: Walter de Gruyter, 1981.

16. von Staden H. "In a pure and holy way": Personal and professional conduct in the Hippocratic Oath. J Hist Med Allied Sci 1996:406–8, contains the *Oath.*

17. Hippocrates: *On Intercourse* [= *Generation*] and *Pregnancy* [= *Nature of the Child*]. Trans. H Ellinger, U Tage. New York: Henry Schuman, 1952.

18. Lefkowitz MR, Fant MB. *Women's Life in Greece and Rome* contains portions of the Hippocratic gynecological treaties using the Littré citation system. These include: *Women's Illnesses* [partial] [*Diseases of Women VIII.12–22, 30–4, 60–2, 64–8, 78, 126.* Tr. Hanson A]; *Displacement of the Womb* [*Places in Human Anatomy V 344–6*]. The dangerous first and sixth forty-day periods during pregnancy [*On the Seventh-Month Child VII 438–42*]. Hysterical suffocation [*Diseases of Women VIII 271–3, 266*]. *Dislocation of the Womb* [*Nature of Women VII 322–4, 314–6*]; and *Hysteria in virgins* [*On Virgins VIII 466–70*]. *www.uky.edu/ ArtsSciences/Classics/wlgr/wlgr-medicine.html*

INDEX TO LOCATION OF HIPPOCRATIC TREATISES

This is an alphabetical list of the location of translations of the Hippocratic Treatises with preference given to titles used in the Loeb editions.

BOOKS

The endnote citation format for books is (Author's last name [year, if not unique] page numbers). I follow the custom of citing quotations from ancient Greek works by line number. Where this is not possible, I note where pages numbers are given.

Adkins AWH. *Merit and Responsibility: A Study in Greek Values.* Oxford: Clarendon Press, 1960.

Aeschylus. *II: The Suppliant Maidens, The Persians, Seven Against Thebes, Prometheus Bound.* Ed. D Grene, R Lattimore. Chicago: University of Chicago Press, 1991.

Aeschylus. *The Oresteia.* Trans. R Fagles. London: Penguin Books, 1966.

Aleshire SB. *The Athenian Asklepieion: The People, Their Dedications, and the Inventories.* Amsterdam: JC Gieben, 1989.

Alic M. *Hypatia's Heritage: A History of Women in Science from Antiquity through the Nineteenth Century.* Boston: Beacon Press, 1986.

Anonymous. *Best of Health: Demographics of Health Care Consumers.* Ithaca: New Strategist Publications, 1998.

Applebaum PS, Lidz CW, Meisel A. *Informed Consent.* Oxford: Oxford University, 1987.

Aristophanes. *Lysistrata, Thesmophoriazusae, Ecclesiazusae, Plutus.* Trans. B Rogers. Vol. III Loeb Classical Library. Cambridge: Harvard University Press, 1988.

Basbanes NA. *A Gentle Madness: Bibliophiles, Bibliomanes, and the Eternal Passion for Books.* New York: Henry Holt, 1995.

Bates D, ed. *Knowledge and the Scholarly Medical Traditions*. Cambridge: Cambridge University Press, 1995.

Beauchamp TL, Childress JF. *Principles of Biomedical Ethics*, 4th ed. New York: Oxford University Press, 1994.

Beauchamp TL, McCullough LB. *Medical Ethics: The Moral Responsibilities of Physicians*. Englewood Cliffs: Prentice-Hall, 1984.

Blundell S. *Women in Ancient Greece*. Cambridge: Harvard University Press, 1995.

Boas G, Cherniss H, Edelstein L, et al. *Studies in Intellectual History*. Baltimore: Johns Hopkins Press, 1953.

Bosk C. *Forgive and Remember*. Chicago: University of Chicago Press, 1979.

Brennan TA. *Just Doctoring: Medical Ethics in the Liberal State*. Berkeley: University of California Press, 1991.

British Medical Association. *Medicine Betrayed: The Participation of Doctors in Human Rights Abuses*. London: Zed Books, 1992.

Brody BA. *Suicide and Euthanasia*. Boston: Kluwer Academic Press, 1989.

Broyard A. *Intoxicated by My Illness*. New York: Fawcett Columbine, 1992.

Bulger RJ, ed. *In Search of the Modern Hippocrates*. Iowa City: University of Iowa Press, 1987.

Calasso R. *The Marriage of Cadmus and Harmony*. New York: Alfred A Knopf, 1993.

Cantarella E. *Bisexuality in the Ancient World*. New Haven: Yale University Press, 1992.

Cantor D, ed. *Reinventing Hippocrates*. Aldershot: Ashgate Publishing, 2002.

Carella MJ. *Matters, Morals and Medicine: The Ancient Greek Origins of Science, Ethics, and the Medical Profession*. New York: Peter Lang Press, 1991.

Carrick P. *Medical Ethics in the Ancient World*. Georgetown: Georgetown University Press, 2001.

Casson L. *Libraries in the Ancient World*. New Haven: Yale University Press, 2001.

Celsus. *De Medicina: Books I–IV*. Trans. WG Spencer. Cambridge: Harvard University Press, 1971.

Childress JF, MacQuarrie J, eds. *Westminister Dictionary of Christian Ethics*. Philadelphia: The Westminister Press, 1967.

Churchill LR. *Self Interest and Universal Health Care*. Cambridge: Harvard University Press, 1994.

Cohen D. *Law, Sexuality, and Society*. Cambridge: Cambridge University Press, 1991.

Cohen D. *Law, Violence and Community in Classical Athens*. Cambridge: Cambridge University Press, 1995.

Committee on Quality of Health Care in America, Kohn LT, et al., eds. *To Err Is Human: Building a Safer Health System*. Washington, D.C.: Institute of Medicine, 2000.

Committee on Understanding and Eliminating Racial and Ethnic Disparities in Health Care, Board on Health Sciences Policy, Institute of Medicine. BD Smedley, AY Stith, AR Nelson, eds., *Unequal Treatment: Confronting Racial and Ethnic Disparities in Health Care.* Washington, D.C.: National Academy Press, 2003.

Copeland L, Lamm LW, eds. *The World's Greatest Speeches.* New York: Dover Publications, 1942.

Ctesias. *La Pers. Linde.* Trans. R Henry, Bruxelles: Office de Publicité, 1947.

Dante Alighieri. *The Portable Dante.* Trans. L Binyon. New York: Viking Press, 1947.

Demand N. *Birth, Death, and Motherhood in Classical Greece.* Baltimore: Johns Hopkins University Press, 1994.

Dodds ER. *The Greeks and the Irrational.* Berkeley: University of California Press, 1964.

Dover KJ. *Greek Homosexuality.* Cambridge: Harvard University Press, 1978.

Edelstein EJ, Edelstein L. *Asclepius: A Collection and Interpretation of the Testimonies.* Baltimore: Johns Hopkins Press, 1945.

Eliade M. *The Sacred and the Profane.* New York: Harper and Row Publishers, 1957.

Englehardt HT. *The Foundations of Bioethics.* New York: Oxford University Press, 1986.

Entralgo L. *The Therapy of the Word in Classical Antiquity.* Trans. LJ Rather, JM Sharp. New Haven: Yale University Press, 1970.

Euripides. *Euripides I: Alcestis, The Medea, The Heracleidae, Hippolytus.* Ed. D Grene, R Lattimore. New York: Washington Square Press, 1955.

Euripides. *Euripides III: Hecuba, Andromache, The Trojan Women, Ion.* Ed. D Grene, R Lattimore Chicago: University of Chicago Press, 1958.

Euripides. *Medea and Other Plays (Medea, Hecabe, Electra, and Heracles).* Trans. P Vellacott. London: Penguin Classics, 1963.

Euripides. *Bacchae and Other Plays: Iphigenia among the Taurians, Bacchae, Iphigenia at Aulis, Rhesus.* Trans. J Morwood. Oxford: Oxford University Press, 1999.

Faden RR, Beauchamp TL. *A History and Theory of Informed Consent.* New York: Oxford University Press, 1986.

Flashar H, Jouanna J. *Médicine et morale dans l'antiquité.* Geneva: Vandoevres, 1996.

Gillespie CC. *Dictionary of Scientific Biography.* New York: Charles Scribners & Sons, 1972.

Fletcher J. *Morals and Medicine.* Boston: Beacon Press, 1954.

Gould SJ. The Mismeasure of Man (rev.). New York, Norton, 1996.

Graves JL. *The Emperor's New Clothes: Biological Theories of Race at the Millennium.* New Brunswick: Rutgers University Press, 2001.

Graves R. *The Greek Myths.* Baltimore: Pelican Books, 1964.

Halperin DM, Winkler JJ, Zeitlin FI, eds. *Before Sexuality: The Construction of Erotic Experience in the Ancient Greek World.* Princeton: Princeton University Press, 1990.

Hastings J. *Encyclopedia of Religion and Ethics.* New York: Charles Scribner & Sons, New York, 1926.

Homer. *The Iliad.* Trans. R Fagles. New York: Penguin Books, 1990.

Horan DJ, Mall D, eds. *Death, Dying, and Euthanasia.* Frederick: Aletheia Books, 1980.

Humez A, Humez N. *Alpha to Omega: The Life and Times of the Greek Alphabet.* Boston: David R Godine Press, 1981.

Hunter KM. *Doctors' Stories: The Narrative Structure of Medical Knowledge.* Princeton: Princeton University Press, 1991.

Irani KD, Silver M. eds. *Social Justice in the Ancient World.* London: Greenwood Press, 1995.

Iserson KV. *Demon Doctors: Physicians as Serial Killers.* Tucson: Galen Press, 2002.

Jonas H. *The Imperative of Responsibility: In Search of an Ethics for the Technological Age.* Chicago: University of Chicago Press, 1984.

Jones WHS. *The Doctor's Oath: An Essay in the History of Medicine.* New York: Cambridge University Press, 1924.

Jones JH. *Bad Blood: The Tuskegee Syphilis Experiment—A Tragedy of Race and Medicine.* New York: Free Press, 1981.

Jonsen AR, Toulmin S. *The Abuse of Casuistry: A History of Moral Reasoning.* Berkeley: University of California Press, 1988.

Jonsen AR. *The Birth of Bioethics.* New York: Oxford University Press, 1998.

Jonsen AR. *A Short History of Medical Ethics.* New York: Oxford University Press, 2000.

Jouanna J. *Hippocrates.* Trans. MB Debevoise. Baltimore: Johns Hopkins Press, 1999.

Kass L. *Toward a More Natural Science: Biology and Human Affairs.* New York: Free Press, 1985.

Katz J. *The Silent World of Doctor and Patient.* New York: Free Press, 1986.

King H. *Hippocrates' Women: Reading the Female Body in Ancient Greece.* London: Routledge Press, 1998.

Kuczewski MG, Polansky R. *Bioethics: Ancient Themes in Contemporary Issues.* Cambridge: MIT Press, 2000.

Langholf V. *Medical Theories in Hippocrates: Early Texts and the "Epidemics."* New York: Walter de Gruyter, 1990.

Lantos J. *Do We Still Need Doctors?* New York: Routledge Publishing, 1997.

Lerner BH. *The Breast Cancer Wars.* New York: Oxford University Press, 2001.

Levi P. *The Periodic Table.* New York: Schocken Books, 1984.

Lifton RJ. *The Nazi Doctors.* New York: Basic Books, 1986.

Lloyd GER. *Magic, Reason, and Experience: Studies in the Origin and Development of Greek Science.* Cambridge: Cambridge University Press, 1979.

Lloyd GER. *Science, Folklore, and Ideology: Studies in the Life Sciences in Ancient Greece*. Cambridge: Cambridge University Press, 1983.

Lloyd GER. *The Revolution in Wisdom: Studies in the Claims and Practice of Ancient Greek Science*. Berkeley: University of California Press, 1987.

Lloyd GER. *Methods and Problems in Greek Science*. Cambridge: Cambridge University Press, 1991.

Lloyd-Jones H. *The Justice of Zeus*. Berkeley: University of California Press, 1983.

Lysias. Trans. WRM Lamb. Cambridge: Loeb Classical Library, 1992.

MacIntyre A. *After Virtue*. Notre Dame: University of Notre Dame Press, 1981.

MacIntyre A. *Whose Justice? Whose Rationality?* Notre Dame: University of Notre Dame Press, 1988.

Majno G. *The Healing Hand: Man and Wound in the Ancient World*. Cambridge: Presidents and Fellows of Harvard College, 1975.

May W. *The Physician's Covenant*. Philadelphia: Westminster Press, 1983.

McMillan RC, Engelhardt HT, Spicker S. *Euthanasia and the Newborn: Conflicts Regarding Saving Lives*. Amsterdam: Dordrecht Press, 1987.

Meier C. *The Greek Discovery of the Polis*. Cambridge: Harvard University Press, 1990.

Mishler EG. *The Discourse of Medicine*. Norwood: Ablex Publishing Company, 1984.

Mundigo AI, Indriso C, eds. *Abortion in the Developing World*. London: Zed Books, 1999.

Murphy LJT. *The History of Urology*. Springfield: Charles C. Thomas, 1972.

Nightingale F. *Notes on Hospitals*. London: Longman, Roberts, and Green, 1863.

Nisbet R. *History of the Idea of Progress*. New York: Basic Books, 1980.

Nussbaum MC. *The Fragility of Goodness: Luck and Ethics in Greek Tragedy and Philosophy*. Cambridge: Cambridge University Press, 1986.

Parker R. *Miasma: Pollution and Purification in Early Greek Religion*. Oxford: Clarendon Press, 1983.

Patterson C. *The Family in Greek History*. Cambridge: Harvard University Press, 1998.

Patterson O. *Freedom in the Making of Western Culture*. New York: Basic Books, 1991.

Pearson L. *Popular Ethics in Ancient Greece*. Stanford University Press, 1962.

Pellegrino E, Thomasma DC. *For the Patient's Good: The Restoration of Beneficence in Health Care*. New York: Oxford University Press, 1988.

Pellegrino E. *Physician Philosopher: The Philosophical Foundation of Medicine: Essays by Dr. Edmund Pellegrino*. Ed. RJ Bulger, JP McGovern. Charlottesville: Carden Jennings Publishing Co., 2001.

Percy W. *The Thanatos Syndrome*. New York: Farrar, Straus, & Giroux, 1987.

Plato. *The Collected Dialogues: Including the Letters*. Ed. E Hamilton, H Cairns. Bollingen Series LXXI, Princeton: Princeton University Press, 1961.

Pomeroy SB. *Goddesses, Whores, and Slaves: Women in Classical Antiquity.* New York: Schocken Books, 1975.

Pomeroy SB. *Women's History and Ancient History.* Chapel Hill: University of North Carolina Press, 1991.

Pomeroy SB. *Families in Classical and Hellenistic Greece.* Oxford: Clarendon Press, 1998.

Potter P, Maloney G, Desautels J. *La maladie et als maladies dans la collection Hippocratique.* Quebec: Editions Sphinx, 1990.

Proctor R. *Racial Hygiene.* Cambridge: Harvard University Press, 1988.

Reich WT, ed. *Encyclopedia of Bioethics.* Revised. New York: Simon and Schuster, Macmillan, 1995.

Robin AE, Key JD. *Medicine Literature and Eponyms.* Malabar, Florida: Robert Krieger, 1989.

Rodwin MA. *Medicine, Money, and Morals: Physicians' Conflicts of Interest.* New York: Oxford University Press, 1993.

Ruse M, ed. *Nature Animated.* Dordrecht: D Reidel Publishing Co., 1983.

Scarborough J, ed. *Folklore and Folk Medicine.* Madison: American Institute of Pharmacy, 1987.

Sealey R. *The Justice of the Greeks.* Ann Arbor: University of Michigan Press, 1997.

Shem S. *The House of God.* New York: Dell Publishing Group, 1979.

Shorter E. *Bedside Manners.* New York: Simon and Shuster, 1985.

Smith WD. *The Hippocratic Tradition.* Ithaca: Cornell University Press, 1979.

Smith WD, ed. and trans. Hippocrates' *Pseudepigraphic Writings: Letters, Embassy, Speech from the Altar, Decree.* New York: Brill Press, 1990.

Sontag S. *Illness as Metaphor.* New York: Farrar, Straus & Giroux, 1977.

Sophocles. *The Three Theban Plays: Antigone, Oedipus the King, Oedipus at Colonus.* Trans. R Fagles, New York: Penguin Books, 1984.

Sophicles. *The Complete Plays.* Trans. P Roche. New York: New American Library, 2001.

Stewart JH. *Analgesic and NSAID-induced Kidney Disease.* New York: Oxford University Press,1993.

Tacitus. *The Annals of Imperial Rome.* Trans. M Grant. New York: Penguin Books, 1956.

Temkin O, Fankena WK, Kadish SH. *Respect for Life in Medicine, Philosophy, and Law.* Baltimore: Johns Hopkins University Press, 1976.

Temkin O, Temkin CL, eds. *Ancient Medicine: The selected papers of Ludwig Edelstein.* Baltimore: Johns Hopkins Press, 1967.

Temkin O. *Hippocrates in a World of Pagans and Christians.* Baltimore: Johns Hopkins University Press, 1991.

Theophrastus. *Enquiry into Plants*. Trans. AF Hort. Cambridge: Harvard University Press, Loeb Classical Library, 1916.

Thomasma DC, Kushner T. *Birth to Death: Science and Bioethics*. Cambridge: Cambridge University Press, 1996.

Thucydides. *The Landmark Thucydides: A Comprehensive Guide to the Peloponnesian War*. Ed. RB Strassler. New York: Simon and Schuster, 1996.

Veatch RM. *A Theory of Medical Ethics*. New York: Basic Books, 1981.

Veatch RM. *The Patient as Partner*. Indianapolis: Indiana University Press, 1987.

Veatch RM, ed. *Cross-Cultural Perspectives in Medical Ethics*, 2nd ed. Boston: Jones and Bartlett Publishers, 2000.

Walzer M. *Spheres of Justice: A Defense of Pluralism and Equality*. New York: Basic Books 1983.

Wangensteen OH, Wangensteen SD. *The Rise of Surgery: From Empiric Craft to Scientific Discipline*. Minneapolis: University of Minnesota Press, 1978.

Wear A. *Medicine in Society: Historical Essays*. Cambridge: Cambridge University Press, 1992.

Weir R, ed. *Physician-Assisted Suicide: Ethical Positions, Medical Practices, and Public Policy Options*. Indianapolis: Indiana Press, 1997.

Wills G. *Lincoln at Gettysburg: The Words That Remade America*. New York: Simon and Schuster, 1992.

Withington ET. *Medical History from the Earliest Times*. London: Holland, 1964.

NOTE

1. Jones (Hippocrates [1923]); Chadwick and Mann (Hippocrates [1950]); Heinrich von Staden, "In a pure and holy way:" Personal and professional conduct in the Hippocratic Oath, J Hist Med Allied Sci 1966;51:406–8.

INDEX